Introduction to Evidence-Based Medicine

Key Summaries for
Common Medical Practices

Introduction to Evidence-Based Medicine

Key Summaries for Common Medical Practices

BLISS CHANG

Harvard Medical School, Class of 2020
Resident in Internal Medicine
New York Presbyterian Hospital
Columbia University
New York City, NY

TIMOTHY FERNANDZ

University of Alabama School of Medicine, Class of 2017
Fellow in Cardiology
Emory University
Atlanta, GA

ELSEVIER

Elsevier
1600 John F. Kennedy Blvd.
Ste 1800
Philadelphia, PA 19103-2899

Notice

Practitioners and researchers must always rely on their own experience and knowledge in evaluating and using any information, methods, compounds or experiments described herein. Because of rapid advances in the medical sciences, in particular, independent verification of diagnoses and drug dosages should be made. To the fullest extent of the law, no responsibility is assumed by Elsevier, authors, editors or contributors for any injury and/or damage to persons or property as a matter of products liability, negligence or otherwise, or from any use or operation of any methods, products, instructions, or ideas contained in the material herein.

Library of Congress Control Number: 2021940079

Content Strategist: Marybeth Thiel
Content Development Specialist: Nicole Congleton
Publishing Services Manager: Deepthi Unni
Project Manager: Haritha Dharmarajan
Design Direction: Margaret Reid

Printed in India

Last digit is the print number: 9   8   7   6   5   4   3   2   1

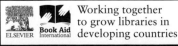

To:

Ahn Hyee and Moon

Nola and Raymond

Thank you for your undying love and support in all that we do.

As a third-year medical student, I found myself wondering why many of the most common practices in medicine were the way they were. I also noticed that there were moments each day where the medical team would have a question about what the evidence was for a particular practice. Furthermore, despite a large movement towards evidence-based medicine over the past few decades, there is not yet an established practice of teaching trainees the evidence behind why they do what they do. And so, this book was born to conveniently empower both early medical trainees as well as more senior medical providers to quickly learn and reference the key evidence driving our everyday actions.

This book focuses on the most common practices that medical trainees will encounter. The evidence presented has been curated carefully with the help of an outstanding group of subspecialty experts at Harvard and Emory-affiliated hospitals. Notably, not all the evidence for any one practice is presented, but rather the most pivotal trials in defining our everyday practices. There are also many helpful practical tips and pointers noted throughout to help early medical trainees build their knowledge base.

Lastly, medical schools continue to ironically dedicate a significant amount of time to teaching students how to dissect basic science research papers. This is a valuable skill that will be utilized by only a tiny percentage of graduating physicians. However, there is not an emphasis on dissecting clinical trials and other studies informing why medicine is practiced the way it is. This is a skill that most physicians use on a routine basis. Thus, this book starts with a short introductory chapter to help those without a statistical background understand enough to interpret clinical studies effectively to inform clinical practice.

Bliss J. Chang, MD
Harvard Medical School
Class of 2020

This book references the key evidence behind the most common medical practices trainees encounter. To facilitate easy navigation, it is divided into medical subspecialties, with each chapter organized by disease and medical practice. Each practice is also associated with key pearls or other practical tips.

For all early trainees, I recommend the following method of utilizing this resource for beginning to learn the evidence behind why you do what you do:

- Begin by reading the Introduction to Evidence-based Medicine chapter for helpful insight into how you should analyze clinical papers and use the evidence presented.
- Focus on broad (e.g., anticoagulation) rather than isolated topics.
- As you learn about the management of various medical conditions throughout your training, try to supplement your learning with this book for a more complete understanding of each case.
- Practice reading the primary source and deriving the same conclusions for each major study as noted in this book.
- Develop a habit of seeking to know what the evidence is for what you're doing.

For medical students, demonstrating your knowledge of the evidence by using it to support your assessment and plans can be very beneficial for both persuading your team of your plan and for earning stellar evaluations. This book serves as a handy reference while you pre-round and assemble your oral presentations. Furthermore, it is a great resource to have at your side for when your team wonders about what the evidence is for a common medical practice. You can greatly help your team by quickly referencing this book.

ADVISORY BOARD

Mark J. Albanese, MD
Assistant Professor of Psychiatry
Harvard Medical School
Boston, MA,
Department of Psychiatry
Cambridge Health Alliance
Cambridge, MA
CHAPTER 11 PSYCHIATRY

Charles J. Grodzin, MD
Assistant Professor
Department of Medicine, Division of
Pulmonary, Allergy, Critical Care, and
Sleep Medicine
Emory University School of Medicine
Atlanta, GA
CHAPTER 3 PULMONOLOGY

Moon Kwoun, MD
Chief of Vascular Surgery, Cambridge Health
Alliance Hospital
Assistant Professor of Medicine, Harvard
Medical School
Boston, MA
CHAPTER 12 VASCULAR MEDICINE & SURGERY

Karen L. Law, MD
Program Director, J. Willis Hurst Internal
Medicine Residency Program
Associate Vice Chair of Education, Emory
University School of Medicine
Associate Professor, Emory University
School of Medicine
Department of Medicine, Division of
Rheumatology
Atlanta, GA
CHAPTER 13 RHEUMATOLOGY

Stewart Lecker, MD, PhD
Assistant Professor of Medicine, Harvard
Medical School
Director, Nephrology Fellowship Training
Program
Beth Israel Deaconess Medical Center
Boston, MA
CHAPTER 6 NEPHROLOGY

**David T. Martin, MD, FRCP, MACP, FACC,
FHRS**
Vice Chair for Network Development and
Innovative Care Solutions
Department of Medicine, Division of
Cardiology
Brigham and Women's Hospital
Boston, MA
CHAPTER 2 CARDIOLOGY

Edison K. Miyawaki, MD
Assistant Professor of Neurology, Harvard
Medical School
Department of Neurology, Brigham and
Women's Hospital
Boston, MA
CHAPTER 5 NEUROLOGY

Bassel Nazha, MD, MPH
Assistant Professor
Department of Hematology and Medical
Oncology, Division of Medical Oncology
Emory University School of Medicine
Atlanta, GA
CHAPTER 7 HEMATOLOGY AND
CHAPTER 8 ONCOLOGY

Emad Qayed, MD, MPH
Associate Professor of Medicine, Emory
University School of Medicine
Chief of Gastroenterology, Grady Memorial
Hospital
Atlanta, GA
CHAPTER 4 GASTROENTEROLOGY

Garrick C. Stewart, MD, MPH
Assistant Professor of Medicine, Harvard
Medical School
Division of Cardiovascular Medicine,
Brigham and Women's Hospital
Boston, MA
CHAPTER 2 CARDIOLOGY

Vin Tangpricha, MD, PhD
Director, Endocrinology Fellowship Training
  Program
Professor, Emory University School of
  Medicine
Department of Medicine, Division of
  Endocrinology
Atlanta, GA
  CHAPTER 10 ENDOCRINOLOGY

Robin Wigmore, MD
Assistant Professor Medicine, Harvard
  Medical School
Department of Infectious Diseases, Beth
  Israel Deaconess Medical Center
Boston, MA
  CHAPTER 9 INFECTIOUS DISEASES

Winona Wu, MD
Integrated Vascular Surgery Resident
Beth Israel Deaconess Medical Center
Boston, MA
  CHAPTER 12 VASCULAR MEDICINE & SURGERY

CONTENTS

Introduction to Evidence-Based Medicine

Approach to Dissecting a Clinical Paper

While each paper can be dissected at great lengths, as a trainee your primary goal is to understand the main results, its implications, and sources of bias. If you can hold a 1000-foot view of these three points, you will be able to begin incorporating evidence-based medicine into your own practice quite soon. Experts will always opine at length on new clinical studies, and it is impractical for you as a young trainee to always do this. The following sections touch upon the core statistical terminology you will encounter, in what we hope is a truly simple manner.

Key Results in a Paper

While there are many results to a paper that can be interesting, here is a short primer on the key results we are most often interested in.

PRIMARY OUTCOMES

Primary outcomes are the key result(s) that the study is designed to investigate. For example, all-cause mortality is a popular primary outcome. Often, the primary outcome is taken as matter of fact, but care should be given to seek context to the outcomes, especially when it is a composite primary outcome.

COMPOSITE OUTCOMES

Very frequently, you will find that the primary outcome is a composite of several outcomes. For example, a study investigating the impact of a new drug on heart failure outcomes may designate its primary outcome as a combination of worsening heart failure or cardiovascular death. These outcomes with more than one outcome are known as composite outcomes. Combining several outcomes, known as end points, allows for a study to be carried out for shorter durations and with fewer participants. However, as you might imagine, composite outcomes lead to difficulty interpreting results since it is difficult to know what particular outcome affected the composite outcome the most.

For example, if a trial aims to investigate whether a medication provides a mortality benefit for patients with heart failure, a composite endpoint of worsening heart failure OR cardiovascular death that meets statistical significance could be driven mostly by worsening heart failure. Thus, when interpreting studies with composite outcomes, pay attention to which of the individual endpoints accounted for the majority ("drove") the significant outcome.

SECONDARY OUTCOMES

Secondary outcomes are those results of interest that help provide context to the primary outcome(s). For example, a primary composite outcome could be driven by one of the variables, and analyzing the secondary outcomes can help elucidate what the primary outcome really means.

Key Factors That Affect Study Validity

The completion and dissemination of a study do not guarantee that the results are accurate nor applicable to clinical practice. As a young trainee, you need not worry too much about the circumstances that lead to a study being practice changing. Your goal should be to understand the key trials, which are mostly well-validated and widely accepted, having been scrutinized by a host of experts in each field. However, here are some basic concepts to begin thinking about as you dive into the evidence behind why we practice medicine the way we do.

THE CONTROL

A study can be designed in ways that artificially boost the strength of a treatment. For example, we now have many medications that form the cornerstones of guideline-directed medical therapy in heart failure with reduced ejection fraction. If a study were to test a new medication, both the control and experimental arms should be on the standard of care medications. Otherwise, we do not know that the benefits of this new medication would even exist on top of current guideline-directed medical therapies.

Another common area for confusion is the use of placebo in the control arm. In most cases, a new treatment should ideally be compared to the standard of treatment, rather than a sugar pill. This also ensures that participants are treated ethically, as if a treatment currently exists, it would be unethical to withhold this from participants regardless of the need for a control arm.

FUNDING

While many people discredit studies that have industry funding, the reality is that it is very difficult in most cases to conduct large randomized clinical trials (RCTs) without some form of industry funding. For example, most of the statin trials were done with industry funding. Thus, it is academically dishonest to jump to a negative view of a study simply due to the source of funding. Every study should be evaluated solely based on the merits of its methodologies.

Common Statistical Vocabulary

Now let us delve into some of the most common statistical terminology that you will encounter. These are by no means comprehensive or technical descriptions and have been simplified for the purposes of warmly introducing you to these terms. As you become familiar with the following terms, practice using them in your everyday discussions about various studies in settings such as rounds. This will help bolster your confidence and actively improve your statistical prowess.

STATISTICAL SIGNIFICANCE

Statistical significance, one of the most common phrases you will encounter, is simply whether the result from an experimental group is reliably (reproducibly) different from that of the control group. In other words, a result that is statistically significant can be trusted.

P VALUE

In simple terms, the P value represents the strength of evidence behind a result. The smaller the P value, the stronger the evidence. The most common P value is set at P > .05, which means that in 95% of cases, your results will be true.

CONFIDENCE INTERVAL

The confidence interval (CI) is the range (interval) of values that will most likely encompass the true value of any result. The most common use of this you will encounter is when comparing two conditions (e.g., experiment vs. control) to see if they are significantly different from each other. CIs that do not overlap in any values are considered significantly different.

SENSITIVITY

Think of sensitivity intuitively as the ability of a test to correctly identifying a target (think "it's so sensitive..."). In other words, sensitivity describes how adeptly a test can identify a "true positive." Hence, you would favor tests that are more sensitive when trying to find a target.

SPECIFICITY

Conversely, sensitivity is how well a test can identify a "true negative." A high specificity means that you can be sure that a negative result will be correct. Note that as the specificity increases, the sensitivity tends to decrease, and vice versa.

POSITIVE PREDICTIVE VALUE

It is easy to confuse this term with sensitivity. Whereas sensitivity is a *proportion*, positive predictive value (PPV) is a *probability*. PPV provides information on how likely a positive result is to be true. A high PPV means that you can be sure that a positive result will be correct.

NEGATIVE PREDICTIVE VALUE

Negative predictive value (NPV) is similar to specificity, but again represents a *probability* rather than a proportion. NPV provides a sense of how likely a negative result is true. You "predict" the value of a negative result.

NUMBER NEEDED TO TREAT

The number needed to treat (NNT) is simply the number of patients who need to be given a certain intervention for one patient to benefit. The lower the NNT, the better an intervention since more patients benefit with the same number of interventions.

NUMBER NEEDED TO HARM

The number needed to harm (NNH) is the number of patients that need to be treated for one patient to experience a "harm" (e.g., side effect). The higher the NNH, the better an intervention since fewer patients are harmed for the same number of treatments.

HAZARD RATIO

Hazard ratios (HRs) deal with the probability of an event (often death) at one point in time. An HR of 1 means there is no difference between the control and experimental groups. An HR greater than 1 means there is less survival (more death, i.e., events) in the experimental group, and vice versa.

RELATIVE RISK

This is an intuitive concept. Relative risk (RR) reflects the chances of an outcome in one group compared to another. For example, an RR of 2 means that an outcome is twice as likely in the intervention arm.

ABSOLUTE RISK

The absolute risk (AR) is akin to the total risk. This is often a better marker than RR because it does not disguise the value of an intervention. For example, a medication may decrease the RR of a disease by 400% which seems very impressive, but if the total (absolute) risk of a disease is 1 in a million, then decreasing this by 400% does not have a great clinical application since the disease is already so rare.

INCLUSION CRITERIA

These are criteria that qualify people for a study, similar to the qualifying times required for the Boston Marathon.

EXCLUSION CRITERIA

These are criteria that make a person ineligible to participate in a study, similar to how a felony may exclude one from serving as an FBI agent.

INTENTION-TO-TREAT ANALYSIS

Intention to treat (IIT) considers the original treatment assignment, also known as "intention." This may be incongruent with the true results when there is large crossover between treatment groups throughout the duration of a study.

ON-TREATMENT ANALYSIS

On-treatment (OT) analysis is analyzing data with respect to what actual treatment was received, rather than what was the intended treatment. This is often seen as a means of addressing large crossovers between treatment groups.

Common Study Types

Clinical evidence is derived from several different study types and methodologies. Though we commonly look to RCTs as the gold standard study design, other methodologies have their own merits and provide evidence in many situations where RCTs are not possible or impractical. Here is a short primer on the two most common study types you will encounter.

RANDOMIZED CLINICAL TRIALS

The gold standard of clinical study types, the RCT allows for the most control over the study design. For instance, a clear cause-and-effect relationship can be established by subjecting one group to a treatment and another group acting as the control. Furthermore, differences in study arms are negated by randomization. While RCTs hold a lot of power and high regard, be sure to check the methods as there are many ways to intentionally and unintentionally guide results in a particular direction. For example, in the famous COMET trial comparing carvedilol to metoprolol, there was a significant setup favoring carvedilol (e.g., using a maximum dose of carvedilol vs. low dose of metoprolol).

COHORT STUDY

A cohort study is a type of prospective observational study, meaning that there are no specific interventions. Instead, the focus is on a group of people who have a particular characteristic(s). While these studies are not as robust as RCTs, they provide advantages particularly when ethical standards do not allow for RCTs. For example, an RCT could never be conducted of a group of people who are forced to smoke or not smoke cigarettes. In short, a cohort study is a great choice for assessing the impact of risk factors on disease incidence.

Cardiology

Arrhythmias

ATRIAL FIBRILLATION

Practice

Chronic atrial fibrillation is a well-recognized risk factor for stroke and systemic thromboembolism.

Evidence
- **Source:** The Framingham Study. Wolf PA, Dawber TR, Thomas HE Jr, Kannel WB. Epidemiologic assessment of chronic atrial fibrillation and risk of stroke: the Framingham study. *Neurology.* 1978;28(10):973–7.
- **Takeaways:**
  - Chronic atrial fibrillation was associated with a fivefold increase in stroke risk.
  - Chronic afib associated with rheumatic heart disease had a 17-fold increase in stroke risk.
- **Notes:**
  - Seminal study that not only demonstrated the link between atrial fibrillation and stroke risk, but also called for study of anticoagulation agents for preventing stroke associated with chronic atrial fibrillation

Practice

Stroke risk is commonly calculated using the CHA_2DS_2VASc scoring system and has major implications for decisions toward initiation of anticoagulation therapy.

Evidence
- **Source:** Lip GYH, Nieuwlaat R, Pisters R, et al. Refining clinical risk stratification for predicting stroke and thromboembolism in atrial fibrillation using a novel risk factor-based approach. *Chest.* 2010;137(2):263–72.

- **Source:** Swedish Atrial Fibrillation Cohort Study. Friberg L, Rosenqvist M, Lip GYH. Evaluation of risk stratification schemes for ischaemic stroke and bleeding in 182 678 patients with atrial fibrillation: the Swedish Atrial Fibrillation cohort study. *Eur Heart J.* 2012;33(12):1500–10.
- **Takeaways:**
  - Improved predictive value of CHA_2DS_2VASc over the CHADS2 score for stroke and thromboembolism
- **Notes:**
  - A recent study (Nielsen PB et al., Circulation 2018) calls into question the role of sex in the scoring scheme and makes a push for determining initial anticoagulation without its use.

Practice

Atrial fibrillation may be controlled with either rate or rhythm control strategies, but rate control is often favored.

Evidence

- **Source:** AFFIRM Trial. Wyse DG, Waldo AL, DiMarco JP, et al. A comparison of rate control and rhythm control in patients with atrial fibrillation. *N Engl J Med.* 2002;347(23):1825–33.
- **Takeaways:**
  - No mortality difference between rate and rhythm control strategies for atrial fibrillation
    - Trend toward decreased mortality with rate control
  - More adverse effects in rhythm-control group
- **Notes:**
  - Rate control may offer advantages such as drugs with fewer side effects, and is typically the first tried method by most clinicians for run of the mill atrial fibrillation.

Practice

Atrial fibrillation in patients with HF with reduced ejection fraction (HFrEF; EF <35%) may be controlled with either rate or rhythm, but rate control is often favored first.

Evidence

- **Source:** AF-CHF Trial. Roy D, Talajic M, Natte S, et al. Rhythm control versus rate control for atrial fibrillation and heart failure. *N Engl J Med.* 2008;358(25):2667–77.
- **Takeaways:**
  - No difference in cardiovascular mortality with rate versus rhythm control
- **Notes:**
  - Rhythm control is pursued if rate control is ineffective in patients with afib and HFrEF.

Practice

Rate control is equal to rhythm control in atrial fibrillation status post cardiac surgery.

Evidence

- **Source:** CTSN Trial. Gillinov AM, Bagiella E, Moskowitz AJ, et al. Rate control versus rhythm control for atrial fibrillation after cardiac surgery. *N Engl J Med.* 2016;374:1911–21.
- **Takeaways:**
  - No significant difference in hospital days and persistent atrial fibrillation at 60 days between rate and rhythm control

- **Notes:**
  - Postoperative atrial fibrillation is typically transient and worst 2 to 4 days after surgery.

Practice

The target heart rate for patients with atrial fibrillation is less than 110 bpm.

Evidence
- **Source:** RACE II Trial. Van Gelder IC, Groenveld HF, Crijns HJGM, et al. Lenient versus strict rate control in patients with atrial fibrillation. *N Engl J Med.* 2010;362(15):1363–73.
- **Takeaways:**
  - No difference in cardiovascular events between strict (<80 bpm) and lenient (<110 bpm) rate control
- **Notes:**
  - Many advantages to lenient rate control!
    - Less stringent outpatient follow-up
    - Less medication/side effects

Practice

Patients with acute (<48 hours) onset atrial fibrillation commonly undergo immediate cardioversion.

Evidence
- **Source:** RACE 7 ACWAS Trial. Pluymaekers NAHA, Dudink EAMP, Luermans JGLM, et al. Early or delayed cardioversion in recent-onset atrial fibrillation. *N Engl J Med.* 2019;380:1499–508.
- **Takeaways:**
  - Delayed cardioversion was noninferior to early cardioversion for achieving sinus rhythm at 4 weeks.
- **Notes:**
  - Delayed cardioversion = initial rate-control strategy with cardioversion after 48 hours if necessary
  - Early cardioversion was done primarily pharmacologically with preference to flecanide.
  - Electrical cardioversion performed when pharmacologic cardioversion contraindicated or prior failure

Practice

The pulmonary veins play a prominent role in the pathogenesis of atrial fibrillation and are often considered for ablation therapy.

Evidence
- **Source:** Haissaguerre M, Jaïs P, Shah DC, et al. Spontaneous initiation of atrial fibrillation by ectopic beats originating in the pulmonary veins. *N Engl J Med.* 1998;339(10):659–66.
- **Takeaways:**
  - 94% of foci identified in afib patients were in the pulmonary veins.
  - 62% of patients with pulmonary vein isolation had no recurrence of afib at follow-up of 8+ months.
- **Notes:**
  - This is the original article that sparked interest in pulmonary vein isolation for treatment of afib!

Practice

In patients without HFrEF who are not symptomatically controlled with antiarrhythmic therapy, pulmonary vein isolation (PVI) is the treatment of choice.

Evidence

- **Source:** CABANA Trial. Packer DL, Mark DB, Robb RA, et al. Effect of catheter ablation vs antiarrhythmic drug therapy on mortality, stroke, bleeding, and cardiac arrest among patients with atrial fibrillation: the CABANA randomized clinical trial. *JAMA*. 2019;321(13):1261–74.
- **Takeaways:**
  - At 1 year, no difference in mortality, bleeding, disabling stroke, or cardiac arrest between PVI and medical therapy
  - 28% greater reduction in atrial fibrillation recurrence with PVI
- **Notes:**
  - The pulmonary veins are the most common foci generating sporadic electrical activity in paroxysmal atrial fibrillation.
  - Persistent atrial fibrillation often occurs from multiple foci and is less amenable to PV isolation.
  - No significant benefit found to adenosine-guided catheter ablation of PVs

Practice

Catheter ablation for atrial fibrillation is preferred over medical therapy in patients with HFrEF (EF <= 35%).

Evidence

- **Source:** AATAC Trial. Di Biase L, Mohanty P, Mohanty S, et al. Ablation versus amiodarone for treatment of persistent atrial fibrillation in patients with congestive heart failure and an implanted device: results from the AATAC multicenter randomized trial. *Circulation*. 2016;133(17):1637–44.
- **Takeaways:**
  - PVI is superior (70%) to medical therapy (34%) for long term maintenance of sinus rhythm.
  - 10% absolute reduction in mortality with PVI
  - 26% absolute reduction in hospitalizations with PVI
- **Source:** CASTLE-AF Trial. Marrouche NF, Brachmann J, Andresen D, et al. Catheter ablation for atrial fibrillation with heart failure. *N Engl J Med* 2018;378(5):417–27.
- **Takeaways:**
  - 11.6% absolute reduction in mortality with catheter ablation
  - 15.2% absolute reduction in HF exacerbation hospitalization
  - 8% versus 0.2% improvement in left ventricular ejection fraction (LVEF) with ablation versus medical therapy
  - 63.1% of ablation and 21.7% of medically treated patients were in sinus rhythm at 60-month follow-up.
- **Notes:**
  - Unclear regarding medical therapy adherence within 60-month follow-up period

Practice

Left atrial appendage (LAA) closure with the WATCHMAN device is an alternative to anticoagulation in patients with nonvalvular afib and high risk of stroke.

Evidence

- **Source:** PROTECT AF Trial. Holmes DR, Reddy VY, Turi ZG, et al. Percutaneous closure of the left atrial appendage versus warfarin therapy for prevention of stroke in patients with atrial fibrillation: a randomised non-inferiority trial. *Lancet.* 2009;374(9689):534–42.
- **Takeaways:**
  - LAA closure was noninferior to warfarin for preventing vascular events (stroke, cardiovascular death, systemic embolism).
  - Higher rate of adverse events driven by periprocedural complications
- **Notes:**
  - Left atrial appendage is the most common location for clots in non-valvular afib.
  - Feasible alternative in patients who are poor anticoagulation candidates

Practice

Under expert judgment, patients on warfarin may not need bridging with low molecular weight heparin (LMWH) for invasive procedures.

Evidence

- **Source:** BRIDGE Trial. Douketis JD, Spyropoulos AC, Kaatz S, et al. Perioperative bridging anticoagulation in patients with atrial fibrillation. *N Engl J Med.* 2015;373(9):823–33.
- **Takeaways:**
  - No LMWH bridge was noninferior (0.4% vs. 0.3%) to perioperative bridging for the prevention of arterial thromboembolism.
  - No LMWH decreased risk of major bleeding.
- **Notes:**
  - LMWH should not be used in patients with severe CKD.

Practice

Aspirin and warfarin are two commonly used agents to reduce risk of stroke, depending on stroke risk as classified by the $CHADS_2VASc$ score.

Evidence

- **Source:** SPAF Trial. SPAF Investigators. Stroke Prevention in Atrial Fibrillation study. *Circulation.* 1991;84(2):527–39.
- **Takeaways:**
  - In nonvalvular atrial fibrillation, aspirin and warfarin both reduced rate of ischemic stroke and systemic embolism.
  - Magnitude of reduction in events on warfarin versus aspirin could not be directly compared.
- **Notes:**
  - First study to investigate the effect of blood thinners and anticoagulants on reducing stroke risk

Practice

Patients at high risk for vascular events such as stroke are anticoagulated.

Evidence

- **Source:** ACTIVE W Trial. Connolly SJ, Pogue J, Hart R, et al. Clopidogrel plus aspirin versus oral anticoagulation for atrial fibrillation in the Atrial fibrillation Clopidogrel Trial with Irbesartan for prevention of Vascular Events (ACTIVE W): a randomised controlled trial. *Lancet.* 2006;367(9526):1903–12.

- **Takeaways:**
  - Warfarin was superior (1.67% absolute risk reduction) to clopidogrel plus aspirin for prevention of vascular events in patients with atrial fibrillation.
  - Similar rates of bleeding between warfarin and dual antiplatelet therapy
- **Notes:**
  - Warfarin is best reversed with fresh frozen plasma (FFP) or cryoprecipitate
  - Vitamin K may be administered but its effects take days

Practice

Dual antiplatelet therapy may be considered for high-risk patients with atrial fibrillation who cannot tolerate anticoagulation.

Evidence

- **Source:** ACTIVE A Trial. Connolly SJ, Pogue J, Hart RG, et al. Effect of clopidogrel added to aspirin in patients with atrial fibrillation. *N Engl J Med.* 2009;360(20):2066–78.
- **Takeaways:**
  - In patients not suited for vitamin-K antagonist anticoagulation, addition of clopidogrel to aspirin reduced rates of major vascular events, particularly stroke.
  - Increased rate of major bleeding (2.0% vs. 1.6%) with dual therapy
- **Notes:**
  - Consider direct oral anticoagulants (DOACs) if warfarin is not tolerated.

Practice

Apixaban is a reasonable alternative for anticoagulation in patients who cannot tolerate warfarin.

Evidence

- **Source:** AVERROES Trial. Connolly SJ, Eikelboom J, Joyner C, et al. Apixaban in patients with atrial fibrillation. *N Engl J Med.* 2011;364(9):806–17.
- **Takeaways:**
  - Apixaban was superior to aspirin in reducing risk of stroke or systemic embolism in patients with atrial fibrillation.
  - No increased bleeding risk compared to aspirin
- **Notes:**
  - Prior to this study, patients who were not warfarin candidates were managed with antiplatelet therapy, either aspirin monotherapy or dual combination with clopidogrel.

Practice

Apixaban is first line for anticoagulation in patients with atrial fibrillation at high risk for stroke.

Evidence

- **Source:** ARISTOTLE Trial. Granger CB, Alexander JH, McMurray JJV, et al. Apixaban versus warfarin in patients with atrial fibrillation. *N Engl J Med.* 2011; 365(11):981-982.
- **Takeaways:**
  - Apixaban was superior (1.27% vs. 1.60%) to warfarin in reducing stroke or systemic embolism.
  - Apixaban resulted in slightly lower mortality (3.52% vs. 3.94%).
  - Apixaban had lower major bleeding risk (2.13% vs. 3.09%).

- **Notes:**
  - Apixaban has the least renal clearance among the DOACs.
  - Apixaban dosing should be reduced to 2.5 mg BID for patients 80+ years, Cr >=1.5, or body weight <= 60 kg.

Practice

Rivaroxaban is a reasonable alternative to warfarin for anticoagulation in patients with atrial fibrillation at high risk for vascular events.

Evidence
- **Source:** ROCKET-AF Trial. Patel MR, Mahaffey KW, Garg J, et al. Rivaroxaban versus warfarin in nonvalvular atrial fibrillation. *N Engl J Med.* 2011;365(10):883–91.
- **Takeaways:**
  - Rivaroxaban was noninferior to warfarin in reducing stroke in nonvalvular atrial fibrillation.
  - No significant difference in bleeding risk
  - Intracranial and fatal bleeding less in rivaroxaban arm
- **Notes:**
  - Among the DOACs, rivaroxaban is convenient because of its once daily dosing.

Practice

Dabigatran is a reasonable alternative to warfarin for anticoagulation in patients with atrial fibrillation at high risk for vascular events.

Evidence
- **Source:** RE-LY Trial. Connolly SJ, Ezekowitz MD, Yusuf S, et al. Dabigatran versus warfarin in patients with atrial fibrillation. *N Engl J Med.* 2009;361:1139–51.
- **Takeaways:**
  - High-dose (110 mg) dabigatran noninferior to warfarin for reducing risk of stroke and systemic embolism
  - Dabigatran had lower risk of major bleeding.
- **Notes:**
  - Dabigatran's antidote is idaricizumab.
  - Do not use dabigatran in presence of mechanical heart valve(s).

Practice

Edoxaban is a reasonable choice for anticoagulation in atrial fibrillation with high risk for stroke.

Evidence
- **Source:** ENGAGE AF-TIMI 48 Trial. Giugliano RP, Ruff CT, Braunwald E, et al. Edoxaban versus warfarin in patients with atrial fibrillation. *N Engl J Med.* 2013;369(22):2093–104.
- **Takeaways:**
  - Edoxaban was noninferior to warfarin in reducing risk of stroke and systemic embolism.
  - Edoxaban was associated with lower bleeding risk.
- **Notes:**
  - Glomerular filtration rate must be between 50 and 95 mL/min per Cockcroft-Gault equation (higher rate of ischemic stroke).

Practice

Patients with atrial fibrillation should be anticoagulated without concomitant aspirin use, without specific indications such as coronary artery disease (CAD).

Evidence

- **Source:** ORBIT-AF Trial. Steinberg BA, Kim S, Piccini JP, et al. Use and associated risks of concomitant aspirin therapy with oral anticoagulation in patients with atrial fibrillation. *Circulation.* 2013;128(7):721–28.
- **Takeaways:**
  - Increased bleeding (3.0% vs. 1.8%) with aspirin therapy on top of anticoagulation
  - Some indication that patients with CAD may benefit from combined therapy with aspirin for reducing future vascular events and death
- **Notes:**
  - 6%-9% of patients were on dabigatran for anticoagulation.

Practice

In patients with atrial fibrillation, triple therapy is recommended after placement of a drug-eluting stent. Providers vary in duration of triple therapy, but growing evidence supports shorter courses (as little as a month).

Evidence

- **Source:** ISAR-TRIPLE Trial. Fiedler KA, Maeng M, Mehilli J, et al. Duration of triple therapy in patients requiring oral anticoagulation after drug-eluting stent implantation: the ISAR-TRIPLE trial. *J Am Coll Cardiol.* 2015;65(16):1619–30.
- **Takeaways:**
  - Six weeks of triple therapy was noninferior to 6 months (9.8% vs. 8.8% in primary endpoint of death, myocardial infarction (MI), stent thrombosis, stroke, or major bleeding).
- **Notes:**
  - Triple therapy = oral anticoagulation + dual antiplatelet therapy
  - If patient has an aspirin allergy and was desensitized for the current admission, it may be wise to continue the aspirin in the case of very high bleeding risk and discontinue the clopidogrel, so that patient is able to continue taking aspirin including in cases of acute MI, without need for re-de-sensitization.

Practice

Andexanet alfa is used as a reversal antidote to apixaban and rivaroxaban.

Evidence

- **Source:** ANNEXA Trial. Siegal DM, Curnutte JT, Connolly SJ, et al. Andexanet alfa for the reversal of factor xa inhibitor activity. *N Engl J Med.* 2015;373:2413–24.
- **Takeaways:**
  - Andexanet reversed the anticoagulant effects of apixaban and rivaroxaban within minutes.
  - No clear evidence of immediate side effects
- **Notes:**
  - Mechanism is binding to the DOAC as a decoy receptor
  - Common andexanet alfa side effects
    - Urinary tract infection
    - Pneumonia

Practice

Prolonged cardiac rhythm monitoring for atrial fibrillation is recommended after cryptogenic stroke.

Evidence
- **Source:** EMBRACE Trial. Gladstone DJ, Spring M, Dorian P, et al. Atrial fibrillation in patients with cryptogenic stroke. *N Engl J Med.* 2014;370(26):2467–77.
- **Takeaways:**
  - 30-day monitoring (16.1%) superior to 24-hour Holter (3.2%) in detecting atrial fibrillation
- **Source:** Dahal K, Chapagain B, Maharjan R, et al. Prolonged cardiac monitoring to detect atrial fibrillation after cryptogenic stroke or transient ischemic attack: a meta-analysis of randomized controlled trials. *Ann Noninvasive Electrocardiol.* 2016;21(4):382–8.
- **Takeaways:**
  - Significantly higher (13.8% vs. 2.5%) detection of atrial fibrillation after cryptogenic stroke with prolonged monitoring (7+ days)
  - Patients who underwent prolonged monitoring were more likely to be anticoagulated at follow-up.
  - No difference in stroke recurrence or mortality
- **Notes:**
  - Patients with an initial cryptogenic stroke are often put on antiplatelet agents rather than anticoagulation during the prolonged monitoring period.

Practice

The Apple Watch is an interesting new development in widely available technology that can alert patients to simple irregular rhythms such as atrial fibrillation.

Evidence
- **Source:** Apple Heart Study. Perez MV, Mahaffey KW, Hedlin H, et al. Large-scale assessment of a smartwatch to identify atrial fibrillation. *N Engl J Med.* 2019;381:1909–17.
- **Takeaways:**
  - 84% of notifications indicating an irregular rhythm were consistent with atrial fibrillation on subsequent ECG.
- **Notes:**
  - This study was also quite monumental in that it was siteless, meaning no hospital visits were required for participants. This type of study supports many future study possibilities, from topics such as adherence, to designs such as effective off-site trials.
  - See editorial: "Watching for Disease: the Changing Paradigm of Disease Screening in the Age of Consumer Health Devices" by David T. Martin and colleagues.

ATRIAL FLUTTER

Practice

The gold standard definitive treatment for typical atrial flutter is cavotricuspid isthmus (CTI) ablation.

Evidence
- **Source:** Perez FJ, Schubert CM, Parvez B, et al. Long-term outcomes after catheter ablation of cavo-tricuspid isthmus dependent atrial flutter. *Circ Arrhythm Electrophysiol.* 2009;2:393–401.
- **Takeaways:**
  - CTI ablation was ~90% successful for typical atrial flutter.
  - ~1/3 of patients took antiarrhythmic drugs after atrial flutter ablation, largely due to new atrial fibrillation post-ablation.

- **Notes:**
  - Atypical atrial flutter typically arises from scarring of the myocardium secondary to procedures/surgery.

ATRIOVENTRICULAR BLOCK

Practice

Single versus dual-chamber pacing for atrioventricular (AV) block is equivocal for the treatment of high-grade AV block in elderly patients (70+ years).

Evidence
- **Source:** UKPACE Trial. Toff WD et al. Single-chamber versus dual-chamber pacing for high-grade atrioventricular block. *N Engl J Med.* 2005;353:145–55.
- **Takeaways:**
  - No difference in mortality or rate of cardiovascular events between single and dual-chamber pacing in elderly patients with high-grade AV block
- **Notes:**
  - Dual chambers are distinct from biventricular pacers—dual chamber refers to pacing of the atrium and ventricle.
  - Dual chamber pacing preserves AV synchrony.

Practice

Dual-chamber pacing offers the option to minimize chronic ventricular pacing and is often preferred, particularly in patients with existing ventricular dysfunction.

Evidence
- **Source:** MOST Trial. Lamas GA, Lee KL, Sweeney MO, et al. Ventricular pacing or dual-chamber pacing for sinus-node dysfunction. *N Engl J Med.* 2002;346(24):1854–62.
- **Takeaways:**
  - Compared to single-chamber pacing, dual-chamber pacing does not lower mortality or stroke.
  - Dual-chamber pacing was associated with a significantly reduced rate of atrial fibrillation (~21.4% vs. 27.1%).
  - Dual-chamber pacing resulted in a small decrease in heart failure hospitalizations.
- **Notes:**
  - Generally, ventricular pacing should be minimized as chronic ventricular pacing leads to increased risk of pacemaker cardiomyopathy (in particular, ventricular dysfunction).

Practice

More and more evidence is pointing toward use of biventricular pacing for AV block with NYHA class I to III heart failure (LVEF <= 50%).

Evidence
- **Source:** BLOCK-HF Trial. Curtis AB, Worley SJ, Adamson PB, et al. Biventricular pacing for atrioventricular block and systolic dysfunction. *N Engl J Med.* 2013;368(17):1585–93.
- **Takeaways:**
  - Biventricular pacing was superior to right ventricular pacing.
  - 9.8% decrease in primary outcome of mortality, urgent care visit for heart failure requiring IV therapy, or increase in LV end-systolic volume index
- **Notes:**
  - 6.4% of patients had LV lead-related complications.

VENTRICULAR ARRHYTHMIAS/SUDDEN CARDIAC DEATH

Practice

In patients with ischemic cardiomyopathy and an implantable cardioverter debrillator (ICD) with persistent ventricular tachycardia despite antiarrhythmic therapy, catheter ablation of arrhythmogenic substrate may be considered over escalating antiarrhythmic dosing.

Evidence
- **Source:** VANISH Trial. Sapp JL, Wells GA, Parkash R, et al. Ventricular tachycardia ablation versus escalation of antiarrhythmic drugs. *N Engl J Med.* 2016; 375:111–21.
- **Takeaways:**
  - Examined patients with ischemic cardiomyopathy and an ICD with ventricular tachycardia despite antiarrhythmic therapy
  - Catheter ablation had significantly lower mortality, ventricular tachycardia storm, or appropriate ICD shock.
- **Notes:**
  - Significant toxicities occurred in the drug (amiodarone) escalation group.

Practice

Prophylactic catheter ablation of arrhythmogenic ventricular tissue may be considered to reduce the incidence of ICD shocks in patients with a history of MI.

Evidence
- **Source:** Reddy VY et al. Prophylactic catheter ablation for the prevention of defibrillator therapy. *N Engl J Med.* 2007;357:2657–65.
- **Takeaways:**
  - Prophylactic substrate-based ablation reduced ICD shocks in patients with ICDs for prevention of sudden cardiac death (SCD) s/p MI.
- **Notes:**
  - ICD shocks are extremely painful and patients may not uncommonly develop psychological consequences (e.g., post-traumatic stress disorder).

Practice

ICD is not recommended early (within 40 days) after an MI for the prevention of SCD.

Evidence
- **Source:** IRIS Trial. Steinbeck G, Andresen D, Seidl K, et al. Defibrillator implantation early after myocardial infarction. *N Engl J Med.* 2009;361:1427–36.
- **Takeaways:**
  - Prophylactic ICD did not reduce mortality in patients with recent MI.
  - Prophylactic ICD had less SCD but greater non-sudden cardiac deaths.
- **Notes:**
  - Supports the results of the DINAMIT trial which showed no benefit to early ICD post-MI

Practice

Prophylactic ICD is not recommended in patients with symptomatic nonischemic HFrEF.

Evidence
- **Source:** DANISH Trial. Kober L, Thune JJ, Nielsen JC, et al. Defibrillator implantation in patients with nonischemic systolic heart failure. *N Engl J Med.* 2016;375:1221–30.

- **Takeaways:**
  - No significant decrease in mortality with prophylactic ICD in symptomatic nonischemic HFrEF
- **Notes:**
  - This is the second major trial to examine ICD use in nonischemic systolic HF; the other is the SCD-HeFT.

Practice

ICD is recommended in patients 40+ days post-MI with HFrEF (LVEF <=35%) and mild to severe symptoms based on expected survival.

Evidence
- **Source:** SCD-HeFT Trial. Bardy GH, Lee KL, Mark DB, et al. Amiodarone or an implantable cardioverter–defibrillator for congestive heart failure. *N Engl J Med.* 2005;352:225–37.
- **Takeaways:**
  - Shock-only ICD therapy decreased mortality by 23%.
  - Amiodarone did not decrease mortality.
- **Notes:**
  - Refer to MADIT trial (in HF section) which preceded this trial

Practice

ICD shocks may provide prognostic information for patients with heart failure.

Evidence
- **Source:** Poole JE, Johnson GW, Hellkamp AS, et al. Prognostic importance of defibrillator shocks in patients with heart failure. *N Engl J Med.* 2008;359:1009–17.
- **Takeaways:**
  - Patients receiving ICD shocks for any arrhythmia had a marked increase in mortality (hazard ratio 5.68 for appropriate shock, 1.98 for inappropriate shock).
- **Notes:**
  - Most common cause of death among patients receiving any shock was progressive heart failure.

OTHER ARRHYTHMIAS

Practice

Physical vagal maneuvers such as carotid massage and Valsalva maneuver are frequently first line for terminating acute symptomatic atrioventricular re-entrant tachycardia (AVRT).

Evidence
- **Source:** Mehta D, Wafa S, Ward DE, Camm AJ. Relative efficacy of various physical manoeuvres in the termination of junctional tachycardia. *Lancet.* 1988;1(8596):1181–5.
- **Takeaways:**
  - Vagal maneuvers were highly successful in terminating AVRT (79%) but not AVNRT (27%). Valsalva maneuver was most successful.
  - Physical maneuvers more effective in younger patients (median 30 years).
- **Notes:**
  - A large reason for attempting physical maneuvers is the terrible feeling associated with IV adenosine administration.

Acute Coronary Syndrome and Coronary Artery Disease

PRACTICE

Aspirin is used in patients with acute MI to reduce cardiovascular mortality.

Evidence

- **Source:** ISIS-2 Trial. ISIS-2 (Second International Study of Infarct Survival) Collaborative Group. Randomized trial of intravenous streptokinase, oral aspirin, both, or neither among 17,187 cases of suspected acute myocardial infarction: ISIS-2. *Lancet.* Aug 13, 1988;332(8607):349–60.
- **Takeaways:**
  - Aspirin use reduced the incidence of cardiovascular mortality at 5 weeks by 2.4% (absolute).
  - Interestingly, the benefit of aspirin and streptokinase was almost additive though the bleeding risk was significantly increased.
- **Notes:**
  - No differences in bleeding events occurred between the control group and aspirin group.

PRACTICE

During acute STEMI, clopidogrel is given early in the treatment course.

Evidence

- **Source:** CLARITY-TIMI 28 Trial. Sabatine MS et al. for the Clopidogrel as Adjunctive Reperfusion Therapy (CLARITY)-Thrombolysis in Myocardial Infarction (TIMI) 28 Investigators. Effect of clopidogrel pretreatment before percutaneous coronary intervention in patients with ST-elevation myocardial infarction treated with fibrinolytics: the PCI-CLARITY study. *JAMA.* Sep 14, 2005;294(10):1224–32.
- **Takeaways:**
  - Clopidogrel pre-treatment group had significantly lower cardiovascular death, reinfarction, or stroke before and after PCI.
  - No differences in bleeding events occurred between the control group and clopidogrel group.
- **Notes:**
  - In patients intolerant to clopidogrel, ticagrelor may be considered with expert evaluation.
  - The rationale for pre-treatment of clopidogrel is to decrease the time to platelet inhibition given that it is first metabolized to its active form in the liver.

PRACTICE

In unstable angina and non-ST segment elevation myocardial infarction (NSTEMI), dual antiplatelet therapy with aspirin and clopidogrel is standard of care for reducing cardiovascular morbidity and mortality in the absence of an indication for coronary artery bypass graft (CABG).

Evidence

- **Source:** CURE Trial. Yusuf S, Zhao F, Mehta SR, et al. Effects of clopidogrel in addition to aspirin in patients with acute coronary syndromes without ST-segment elevation. *N Engl J Med.* Aug 16, 2001;345(7):494–502.

- **Takeaways:**
  - In unstable angina and NSTEMI, use of DAPT resulted in decreased cardiovascular death, nonfatal MI, and stroke compared to aspirin alone.
  - Increased bleeding in patients treated with clopidogrel (1% absolute increase)
- **Notes:**
  - Clopidogrel, and all antiplatelets besides aspirin, requires a loading dose prior to the daily maintenance dose. The loading dose helps to kickstart platelet inhibition at sufficient rates.

PRACTICE

Ticagrelor is preferred over clopidogrel in patients with ACS.

Evidence

- **Source:** PLATO Trial. Wallentin L, Becker RC, Budaj A, et al. Ticagrelor versus clopidogrel in patients with acute coronary syndromes. *N Engl J Med.* Sep 10, 2009;361(11):1045–57.
- **Takeaways:**
  - Ticagrelor outperformed clopidogrel for cardiovascular death, MI, or stroke.
  - No increase in bleeding in the ticagrelor arm compared to clopidogrel
- **Notes:**
  - Ticagrelor is unique as an antiplatelet agent in that it is reversible, as opposed to clopidogrel and prasugrel.

PRACTICE

Prasugrel is an alternative antiplatelet used in patients with ACS.

Evidence

- **Source:** TRITON TIMI-38 Trial. Wiviott SD et al. for the TRITON-TIMI 38 Investigators. Evaluation of prasugrel compared with clopidogrel in patients with acute coronary syndromes: design and rationale for the TRial to assess Improvement in Therapeutic Outcomes by optimizing platelet InhibitioN with prasugrel Thrombolysis in Myocardial Infarction 38 (TRITON-TIMI 38). *Am Heart J.* Oct 2006;152(4):627–35.
- **Takeaways:**
  - Similar to the PLATO trial, prasugrel reduced cardiovascular death, MI, or stroke when compared to clopidogrel.
  - However, unlike PLATO, the incidence of significant bleeding was increased.
- **Notes:**
  - Among the common antiplatelet agents, prasugrel is considered the strongest both in terms of platelet inhibition and bleeding risk.

PRACTICE

In acute myocardial infarction, patients are started on beta-blockers.

Evidence

- **Source:** COMMIT Trial. Chen ZM et al. for the COMMIT (ClOpidogrel and Metoprolol in Myocardial Infarction Trial) collaborative group. Early intravenous then oral metoprolol in 45,852 patients with acute myocardial infarction: randomised placebo-controlled trial. *Lancet.* Nov 5, 2005;366(9497):1622–32.

- **Takeaways:**
  - In the COMMIT treatment, early use of metoprolol, however, decreased the risk of reinfarction and ventricular fibrillation.
  - Slight increase in risk of cardiogenic shock with the use of beta-blockers
- **Notes:**
  - Due to the risk of cardiogenic shock when beta-blockers are applied, patients should be assessed for hemodynamic stability prior to use. Patients at increased susceptibility include those with involvement of the right ventricle.

PRACTICE

After acute myocardial infarction, patients are started on ACE (angiotensin-converting enzyme) inhibitors.

Evidence

- **Source:** SAVE Trial. Pfeffer MA, Braunwald E, Moyé LA, et al. Effect of captopril on mortality and morbidity in patients with left ventricular dysfunction after myocardial infarction. Results of the survival and ventricular enlargement trial. The SAVE Investigators. *N Engl J Med.* Sep 3, 1992;327(10):669–77.
- **Takeaways:**
  - Treating patients with captopril in acute MI with asymptomatic left ventricular dysfunction reduced mortality from cardiovascular causes.
  - The captopril group had lower rates of hospitalization due to heart failure and recurrent MI.
- **Notes:**
  - Captopril is a nice ACE inhibitor to start a patient on during MI due to its short duration of action. It can then be titrated easily to a target daily dose or transitioned to a longer acting ACE inhibitor such as lisinopril.

PRACTICE

In patients with STEMI who presents to centers where PCI is unavailable, inter-hospital transfer for primary PCI is preferred if the transfer time is less than 2 hours.

Evidence

- **Source:** DANAMI-2 Trial. Andersen HR et al. for the DANAMI-2 Investigators. A comparison of coronary angioplasty with fibrinolytic therapy in acute myocardial infarction. *N Engl J Med.* Aug 21, 2003;349(8):733–42.
- **Takeaways:**
  - At percutaneous coronary intervention (PCI)-incapable hospitals, transfer to a PCI-capable center is superior to thrombolysis if the transfer time is under 2 hours.
- **Notes:**
  - If the transfer time is too long, fibrinolytic therapy should be administered within 30 minutes of arrival to the hospital.

PRACTICE

PCI is not performed routinely in patients with stable coronary artery disease.

Evidence

- **Source:** COURAGE Trial. Boden WE et al. for the COURAGE Trial Research Group. Optimal medical therapy with or without PCI for stable coronary disease. *N Engl J Med.* Apr 12, 2007;356(15):1503–16.
- **Takeaways:**
  - No significant difference between medical therapy and PCI in stable coronary artery disease for primary endpoint of death and nonfatal MI
- **Notes:**
  - All patients were optimized on an ACE or ARB, antiplatelet agent, as well as a combination of beta-blockers, calcium channel blockers, and nitrates. All patients also received lipid-lowering agents.

PRACTICE

In patients with multivessel coronary artery disease who are undergoing PCI, the measurement of fractional flow reserve is routinely performed.

Evidence

- **Source:** FAME FFR Trial. Tonino PA et al. for the FAME Study Investigators. Fractional flow reserve versus angiography for guiding percutaneous coronary intervention. *N Engl J Med.* Jan 15, 2009;360(3):213–24.
- **Takeaways:**
  - For multivessel and anatomically complex coronary disease, fractional flow reserve (FFR)-guided PCI compared to routine PCI reduces mortality, nonfatal MI, and revascularization at 1 year.
- **Notes:**
  - FFR is a measurement of the pressure difference across a stenotic region. Thus, it is the ratio of blood flow in the presence of the stenosis compared to the (theoretical) maximal flow without stenosis.

PRACTICE

In diabetic patients with multivessel coronary disease, CABG is the preferred modality for revascularization.

Evidence

- **Source:** FREEDOM Trial. Farkouh ME et al. for the FREEDOM Trial Investigators. Strategies for multivessel revascularization in patients with diabetes. *N Engl J Med.* Dec 20, 2012;367(25):2375–84.
- **Takeaways:**
  - Patients with type 2 diabetes and multivessel CAD saw an 8.1% increase in death, nonfatal MI, or stroke with PCI compared to CABG.
  - CABG was associated with a twofold increase in stroke.

PRACTICE

The radial artery is the preferred access for PCI.

Evidence

- **Source:** RIVAL Trial. Jolly SS et al. for the RIVAL trial group. Radial versus femoral access for coronary angiography and intervention in patients with acute coronary syndromes (RIVAL): a randomised, parallel group, multicentre trial. *Lancet.* Apr 23, 2011;377(9775):1409–20.
- **Takeaways:**
  - No difference in death, myocardial infarction, stroke, and non-CABG-related major bleeding between groups at 30 days
  - However, PCI with radial access had significantly lower rates of vascular complications compared to femoral access.
- **Notes:**
  - Radial access requires the Allen test beforehand to ensure that the patient has collateral circulation to the hand/arm via the ulnar artery.

PRACTICE

In patients with severe coronary artery disease, coronary artery bypass graft surgery should be the standard of care.

Evidence

- **Source:** SYNTAX Trial. Serruys PW et al. for the SYNTAX Investigators. Percutaneous coronary intervention versus coronary-artery bypass grafting for severe coronary artery disease. *N Engl J Med.* Mar 5, 2009;360(10):961–72.
- **Takeaways:**
  - The local cardiac surgeon and interventional cardiologist determined that equivalent anatomical revascularization could be achieved with either PCI or CABG.
  - Rates of major adverse cardiac or cerebrovascular events at 12 months were significantly higher in the PCI group (17.8%, vs. 12.4% for CABG).
  - The primary endpoint was driven by an increased rate of repeat revascularization.
  - Stroke was significantly more likely with CABG.
- **Notes:**
  - The SYNTAX score is a measure of the complexity of the anatomy for a coronary artery lesion. The higher the score, the higher the complexity.

PRACTICE

In patients with known coronary disease, statins are standard of care.

Evidence

- **Source:** CARE Trial. Sacks FM, Pfeffer MA, Moye LA, et al. The effect of pravastatin on coronary events after myocardial infarction in patients with average cholesterol levels. Cholesterol and Recurrent Events Trial investigators. *N Engl J Med.* Oct 3, 1996;335(14):1001–9.
- **Takeaways:**
  - Compared to placebo, statins significantly decreased the risk of cardiovascular events, most notably nonfatal MI.
  - The greater the baseline LDL, the greater the reduction benefit from statins.
- **Notes:**
  - Rosuvastatin is the only renally cleared statin. Adjust the dosing or stick to atorvastatin in patients with CKD or significant acute kidney injury (AKI).

PRACTICE

In patients with a recent acute coronary syndrome, high-intensity statins are started to reduce the risk of recurrent ischemia and reduce mortality.

Evidence

- **Source:** MIRACL Trial. Schwartz GG et al for the Myocardial Ischemia Reduction with Aggressive Cholesterol Lowering (MIRACL) Study Investigators. Effects of atorvastatin on early recurrent ischemic events in acute coronary syndromes: the MIRACL study: a randomized controlled trial. *JAMA.* Apr 4, 2001;285(13):1711–8.
- **Source:** PROVE IT Trial. Cannon CP, Braunwald E, McCabe CH, et al for the Pravastatin or Atorvastatin Evaluation and Infection Therapy-Thrombolysis in Myocardial Infarction 22 Investigators. Intensive versus moderate lipid lowering with statins after acute coronary syndromes. *N Engl J Med.* Apr 8, 2004;350(15):1495–504.
- **Takeaways:**
  - In the MIRACL trial, when atorvastatin 80 mg was initiated in patients with unstable angina or NSTEMI within 24 to 96 hours, there was a significant reduction in death, nonfatal MI, cardiac arrest, and ACS.
  - In the PROVE IT trial, high-dose atorvastatin demonstrated a 16% reduction in death or major cardiovascular event compared to standard moderate-dose pravastatin therapy.
  - The protective effect of intensive lipid-lowering was evident in the first 30 days of therapy and was consistent across pre-specified subgroups.
- **Notes:**
  - Other high-intensity statins include atorvastatin 40 mg, rosuvastatin 20 mg, and rosuvastatin 40 mg. Simvastatin 80 mg was historically a high-intensity dose but retired due to increased rates of rhabdomyolysis.

PRACTICE

In addition to moderate-intensity statins, ezetimibe is used to further reduced LDL cholesterol levels, particularly in the setting of recent ACS.

Evidence

- **Source:** IMPROVE-IT Trial. Cannon CP et al for the IMPROVE-IT Investigators. Ezetimibe added to statin therapy after acute coronary syndromes. *N Engl J Med.* Jun 18, 2015;372(25):2387–97.
- **Takeaways:**
  - The combination of ezetimibe and moderate-intensity simvastatin led to a further decrease in cardiovascular morbidity and mortality of 2% (absolute).
- **Notes:**
  - Although in the trial, a moderate intensity statin was utilized, many patients are on high-intensity statins prior to the start of ezetimibe.

PRACTICE

In patients with CAD (or diabetes and one extra risk factor) and triglyceride levels >135 already on statin therapy, icosapentethyl is used to reduce cardiovascular mortality.

Evidence

- **Source:** REDUCE-IT Trial. Cannon CP et al for the IMPROVE-IT Investigators. Ezetimibe added to statin therapy after acute coronary syndromes. *N Engl J Med.* Jun 18, 2015;372(25):2387–97.
- **Takeaways:**
  - High-dose (4 g/day) icosapentethyl ether reduced cardiovascular death by 0.9% at 5 years when added to statin therapy in patients with triglycerides greater than 135.
- **Notes:**
  - Icosapentethyl ether has come under criticism from some groups for inconsistent results demonstrating cardiovascular benefit. However, trial results are consistent when a high dose (4 g/day) is utilized, with lower dose trials demonstrating lack of benefit.

Heart Failure

Heart failure (HF) comes in several flavors, most prominent of which are HF with reduced ejection fraction (HFrEF) and HF with preserved ejection fraction (HFpEF). To date, the vast majority of evidence for successful therapeutic intervention in heart failure has been specific to HFrEF, with extrapolation of this evidence to its sibling varieties.

HFrEF (CHRONIC MANAGEMENT)

Practice

Patients with HFrEF are prescribed a lifelong course of ACEI/ARBs for their mortality benefits.

Evidence
Angiotensin Converting Enzyme Inhibitors

- **Source:** SAVE Trial. Pfeffer MA, Braunwald E, Moyé LA, et al. Effect of captopril on mortality and morbidity in patients with left ventricular dysfunction after myocardial infarction. Results of the survival and ventricular enlargement trial. *N Engl J Med.* 1992;327(10):669–77.
- **Takeaways:**
  - Absolute all-cause mortality decreased by 5% in patients with EF less than 40% after MI taking ACEI.
  - This set the stage for all the investigations into the RAAS pathway for heart failure therapy.
- **Source:** CONSENSUS Trial. The CONSENSUS Trial Study Group. Effects of enalapril on mortality in severe congestive heart failure. *N Engl J Med.* 1987;316:1429–35.
- **Takeaways:**
  - 18% mortality reduction in HFrEF with NYHA class IV symptoms
- **Notes:**
  - First trial to demonstrate a mortality benefit of any therapeutic agent for HFrEF
- **Source:** SOLVD Trial. The SOLVD Investigators. Effect of enalapril on survival in patients with reduced left ventricular ejection fractions and congestive heart failure. *N Engl J Med.* 1991;325:293–302.
- **Takeaways:**
  - 16% mortality benefit in patients with cardiovascular disease
- **Notes:**
  - First line for all HFrEF patients
  - ACEI/ARBs thought to deter pathologic remodeling of the heart

Angiotensin Receptor Blockers
- **Source:** Val-HeFT Trial. Cohn JN, Tognoni G, Valsartan Heart Failure Trial Investigators. A randomized trial of the angiotensin-receptor blocker valsartan in chronic heart failure. *N Engl J Med.* 2001;345:1667–75.
- **Source:** CHARM Trial. McMurray JJ et al. Effects of candesartan in patients with chronic heart failure and reduced left-ventricular systolic function taking angiotensin-converting-enzyme inhibitors: the CHARM-Added trial. *Lancet.* 2003;362(9386):767–71.
- **Takeaways:**
  - Primary composite endpoint of cardiovascular mortality or hospitalization for heart failure lower with ARB treatment
  - Patients were already on ACE inhibitors; these studies added the ARB on top of the ACEI.
- **Source:** ONTARGET Trial. The ONTARGET Investigators. Telmisartan, ramipril, or both in patients at high risk for vascular events. *N Engl J Med* 2008;358:1547–59.
- **Takeaways:**
  - ARBs noninferior to ACEI in mortality benefit for patients with cardiovascular disease
  - Combination of ACEI + ARB had no increased benefit but had more adverse effects.
- **Notes:**
  - Second-line for HFrEF, only if intolerant of ACEI
  - ACEI/ARBs thought to deter pathologic remodeling of the heart

Practice

For patients intolerant to ACE inhibitors, ARBs are the first-line alternative therapy.

Evidence
- **Source:** CHARM-Alternative Trial. Granger CB, McMurray JJV, Yusuf S, et al. Effects of candesartan in patients with chronic heart failure and reduced left-ventricular systolic function intolerant to angiotensin-converting-enzyme inhibitors: the CHARM-Alternative Trial. *Lancet.* 2003;362(9386):772–6.
- **Takeaways:**
  - 20% cardiovascular mortality benefit with ARB use in patients intolerant to ACEI
  - 40% reduction in heart failure hospitalizations
- **Notes:**
  - First trial to look at using an ARB in lieu of an ACEI (the prior trials were stacking ARBs on top of ACEIs)

Practice

Patients with HFrEF are prescribed a lifelong course of beta-blockers for their mortality benefits. The three with proven benefits are:
- Metoprolol succinate
- Bisoprolol
- Carvedilol

Evidence
Metoprolol Succinate
- **Source:** MERIT-HF Trial. MERIT-HF Study Group. Effect of metoprolol CR/XL in chronic heart failure: Metoprolol CR/XL Randomised Intervention Trial in-Congestive Heart Failure. *Lancet.* 1999;353(9169):2001–7.
- **Takeaways:**
  - 34% reduction in mortality for EF <= 40%

- **Notes:**
  - First-line beta-blocker used for HFrEF
  - Metoprolol tartrate is often used to help fractionate doses and match the hospital drug administration times or to allow flexibility and increased control of drug administration doses/times.
    - Patients should be on metoprolol succinate long term, as metoprolol tartrate has not been explicitly proven yet in a clinical trial to have the same mortality benefit as its succinate counterpart.
  - For heart failure patients, always check medication lists to ensure that the patient is on succinate rather than tartrate when there is not a clear need for tartrate.

Carvedilol
- **Source:** U.S. Carvedilol Trials. Packer M, Bristow MR, Cohn JN, et al. The effect of carvedilol on morbidity and mortality in patients with chronic heart failure. *N Engl J Med.* 1996;334:1349–55.
- **Takeaways:**
  - 4.6% absolute reduction in all-cause mortality in carvedilol group compared to placebo
- **Source:** COPERNICUS Trial. Packer M, Fowler MB, Roecker EB, et al. Effect of carvedilol on the morbidity of patients with severe chronic heart failure: results of the carvedilol prospective randomized cumulative survival (COPERNICUS) study. *Circulation.* 2002;106(17):2194–9.
- **Takeaways:**
  - 31% reduction in mortality and HF exacerbation hospitalization in EF less than 25% and NYHA class III to IV
- **Notes:**
  - First trial to establish the role of beta-blockers in HF with severely reduced EF
  - Second-line beta-blocker used for HFrEF
  - More significant blood pressure–lowering effect than other mortality-reducing beta-blockers due to alpha-1 antagonism

Bisoprolol
- **Source:** CIBIS-II Trial. The SOLVD Investigators. The Cardiac Insufficiency Bisoprolol Study II (CIBIS-II): a randomised trial. *Lancet.* 1999;353:9146:9–13.
- **Takeaways:**
  - 34% reduction in mortality for EF <= 35% and NYHA class III to IV
- **Notes:**
  - Third-line beta-blocker used for HFrEF in the United States; often first line in Europe
  - Bisoprolol is the most cardioselective of the three beta-blockers, often favored when asthma/COPD are present.

Practice

Carvedilol and metoprolol are both viable medications for reducing mortality in HFrEF. Due to study flaws below, it is difficult to say that carvedilol is superior to metoprolol.

Evidence

- **Source:** COMET Trial. Poole-Wilson PA, Swedberg K, Cleland JGF, et al. Comparison of carvedilol and metoprolol on clinical outcomes in patients with chronic heart failure in the Carvedilol Or Metoprolol European Trial (COMET): randomised controlled trial. *Lancet.* 2003;362(9377):7–13.
- **Takeaways:**
  - Carvedilol had a greater mortality benefit than metoprolol tartrate in HFrEF (LVEF <= 35%).

- **Notes:**
  - The trial was heavily biased to favor carvedilol.
    - Max dose of carvedilol versus half-max dose of metoprolol tartrate
    - Metoprolol succinate (not tartrate) was shown to have the mortality benefit in MERIT-HF.
  - Some cardiologists take this to mean that carvedilol is better than metoprolol; however, in our experience, more cardiologists understand this to be a very biased study and choose between metoprolol succinate and carvedilol based on other factors, such as blood pressure (carvedilol has better BP-lowering effects).
  - Guidelines suggest a class effect of beta-blockers.
  - Carvedilol has the greatest blood pressure–lowering effect among the three beta-blockers with mortality benefits.

Practice

Black patients with HFrEF are prescribed a lifelong course of isosorbide dinitrate + hydralazine for their mortality benefits.

Evidence

Isosorbide Dinitrate + Hydralazine
- **Source:** A-HeFT Trial. Taylor AL, Ziesche S, Yancy C, et al. Combination of isosorbide dinitrate and hydralazine in blacks with heart failure. *N Engl J Med.* 2004;351:2049–57.
- **Takeaways:**
  - Mortality benefit and reduced hospitalizations in black patients with HFrEF
- **Notes:**
  - Follow-up to a prior trial V-HeFT where a subgroup analysis demonstrated possible benefit in specifically black patients
  - This increased benefit as opposed to use of ACEI/BBs may be explained by the tendency of black patients to possess less robust RAAS-system activity (upon which ACEI/BB effects depend).
  - Do not use in patients at risk of hypotension.

Practice

In HF patients, Entresto/ARNI is considered as a superior replacement for well-tolerated ACEI/ARB therapy. Current use is limited primarily due to cost, but its use is steadily spreading.

Evidence

Entresto: Sacubitril (Neprilysin inhibitor) + Valsartan (Angiotensin II receptor blocker)
- **Source:** PARADIGM-HF Trial. McMurray JJ, Packer M, Desai AS, et al. Angiotensin–neprilysin inhibition versus enalapril in heart failure. *N Engl J Med.* 2014;371:993–1004.
- **Takeaways:**
  - 19.8% all-cause mortality benefit in HFrEF
  - 26.5% reduction in CV mortality or HF exacerbation hospitalization
- **Notes:**
  - Neprilysin: enzyme that breaks down BNP and bradykinin
  - Long-term side-effect profile unclear
  - Very expensive
  - Do not prescribe if history of ACEI angioedema.
  - Do not prescribe together with ACEIs (must wait 36 hours after previous dose).

Practice

Patients with HFrEF (EF <= 35%) are prescribed a lifelong course of mineralocorticoid receptor antagonists (MRAs) for their mortality benefits.

Evidence
Spironolactone
- **Source:** RALES Trial. Pitt B, Zannad F, Remme WJ, et al. The effect of spironolactone on morbidity and mortality in patients with severe heart failure. *N Engl J Med.* 1999;341:709–717.
- **Takeaways:**
  - 30% reduction in mortality in HFrEF, NYHA class III to IV
- **Notes:**
  - Key side effects include hyperkalemia and gynecomastia (in men).
  - Always check for risk of hyperkalemia.

Epleronone
- **Source:** EPHESUS Trial. Pitt B, Remme W, Zannad F, et al. Eplerenone, a selective aldosterone blocker, in patients with left ventricular dysfunction after myocardial infarction. *N Engl J Med.* 2003;348:1309–21.
- **Takeaways:**
  - Mortality benefit in acute MI with HF symptoms and LV dysfunction
- **Notes:**
  - First evidence for epleronone as a useful alternative in HFrEF for men who experience significant gynecomastia (less anti-androgenic side effects)
- **Source:** EMPHASIS-HF Trial. Zannad F, McMurray JJV, Krum H, et al. Eplerenone in patients with systolic heart failure and mild symptoms. *N Engl J Med.* 2011;364:11–21.
- **Takeaways:**
  - Mortality benefit in HFrEF even with mild symptoms (NYHA class II)
- **Notes:**
  - EMPHASIS-HF suggests that moderate-severe HFrEF of all symptom severities benefit from aldosterone antagonism.

Practice

SGLT2 inhibitors are used for their robust all-cause mortality benefit and reduction in HF hospitalizations in patients with HFrEF.

Evidence
- **Source:** CANVAS Trial. Neal B, Perkovic V, Matthews DR. Canagliflozin and cardiovascular and renal events in type 2 diabetes. *N Engl J Med.* 2017;377:644–57.
- **Takeaways:**
  - 4.4% absolute reduction in cardiovascular mortality in type 2 diabetics
  - Increased risk of toe/metatarsal amputation
- **Source:** DAPA-HF Trial. McMurray JJV, Solomon SD, Inzucchi SE, et al. Dapagliflozin in patients with heart failure and reduced ejection fraction. *N Engl J Med.* 2019;381:1995–2008.
- **Key Criteria:**
  - Inclusion: LVEF <= 40%, ± T2DM
- **Takeaways:**
  - Decreased mortality and risk of worsening HF with SGLT2 inhibitors on top of current goal-directed medical therapy

■ **Notes:**
  ■ The DAPA-HF trial built on the DECLARE-TIMI 58 trial which demonstrated the mortality benefit of SGLT2 inhibitors in HFrEF, but only in type 2 diabetics.
  ■ The interaction between diabetes and HF is complex and continually evolving; prior drug classes have even caused harm (thiazolidinediones)!

Practice

Ivabradine is used for additional symptomatic management in HFrEF in patients already on maximal goal-directed medical therapy with heart rates >70 bpm.

Evidence

■ **Source:** SHIFT Trial. Swedberg K, Komajda M, Böhm M, et al. Ivabradine and outcomes in chronic heart failure (SHIFT): a randomised placebo-controlled study. *Lancet.* 2010;376(10):875–85.
■ **Takeaways:**
  ■ 5% absolute reduction in mortality at 2 years
    Subsequent subgroup analysis revealed little mortality benefit for patients already receiving at least 50% of the intended beta-blocker dosages.
  ■ Ivabradine significantly decreased HF exacerbation hospitalizations.
■ **Notes:**
  ■ Ivabradine works by blocking the funny current.
  ■ Common side effect is luminous phenomena where patients experience increased brightness in their visual field.
  ■ Ivabradine should not be given during acute decompensated heart failure (ADHF).

Practice

Digoxin is used for symptomatic management of HFrEF and to reduce hospitalizations.

Evidence

■ **Source:** DIG Trial. Gorlin R et al. The effect of digoxin on mortality and morbidity in patients with heart failure. *N Engl J Med.* 1997;336(8):525–33.
■ **Takeaways:**
  ■ Digoxin did not reduce mortality in HFrEF.
  ■ Reduced rates of hospitalization
■ **Notes:**
  ■ Digoxin levels must be monitored carefully and are very sensitive to interactions with other medications and overall volume status.
  ■ Hypercalcemia can potentiate digoxin.
  ■ Decrease digoxin levels by approximately 25% to 50% when initiating amiodarone due to drug-drug interactions leading to increased digoxin levels.

Practice

Patients with HFrEF and iron deficiency are supplemented with IV iron for symptomatic management.

Evidence

■ **Source:** FAIR-HF Trial. Anker SD, Comin Colet J, Filippatos G, et al. Ferric carboxymaltose in patients with heart failure and iron deficiency. *N Engl J Med.* 2009;361(25): 2436–48.

- **Takeaways:**
  - Significant increases in symptoms and NYHA functional class
- **Notes:**
  - The definition of iron deficiency in HF differs from other conditions of chronic inflammation and is defined as:
    - Ferritin <100 µg/L, or
    - Ferritin 100 to 299 µg/L with a transferrin saturation of <20%
  - The trial included patients with iron deficiency but mild or no anemia; no patients with significant anemia were included.
  - Although different iron formulations are used, ideally should be ferric carboxymaltose

Practice

ICD is recommended for its mortality benefit in patients 40+ days post-MI with HFrEF (LVEF <=35%) and mild to severe symptoms based on expected survival.

Evidence

- **Source:** MADIT-II Trial. Moss AJ, Zareba W, Hall WJ, et al. Prophylactic implantation of a defibrillator in patients with myocardial infarction and reduced ejection fraction. *N Engl J Med.* 2002;346(12):877–83.
- **Takeaways:**
  - 5.6% decrease in all-cause mortality with prophylactic ICD implantation
  - Patient population had EF <=30%.
- **Source:** SCD-HeFT Trial. Bardy GH, Lee KL, Mark DB, et al. Amiodarone or an implantable cardioverter–defibrillator for congestive heart failure. *N Engl J Med.* 2005;352:225–37.
- **Takeaways:**
  - Shock-only ICD therapy decreased mortality by 23%.
  - Amiodarone did not decrease mortality.
- **Source:** DEFINITE Trial. Prophylactic defibrillator implantation in patients with non-ischemic dilated cardiomyopathy. *N Engl J Med.* 2004;350(21):2151–8.
- **Takeaways:**
  - 6.2% absolute reduction in mortality at 2 years in ICD group
  - Significant reduction in sudden death with ICD
- **Notes:**
  - All patients were already on maximal goal-directed medical therapy for HFrEF.

Practice

Cardiac resynchronization therapy (CRT) is recommended in patients with HFrEF (LVEF <= 35%) and QRS >= 120 msec for mortality and symptomatic management.

Evidence

- **Source:** CARE-HF Trial. Cleland JGF, Daubert JC, Erdmann E, et al. The effect of cardiac resynchronization on morbidity and mortality in heart failure. *N Engl J Med.* 2005;352:1539–49.
- **Takeaways:**
  - 10% absolute reduction in mortality with CRT
  - Significant symptomatic improvement with CRT
- **Notes:**
  - CRT by definition includes a pacemaker (often termed CRT-P).

Practice

Patients with QRS >= 130msec and HFrEF (LVEF <= 30%) receive cardiac resynchronization therapy on top of ICD.

Evidence

- **Source:** MADIT-CRT Trial. Moss AJ, Hall WJ, Cannom DS, et al. Cardiac-resynchronization therapy for the prevention of heart-failure events. *N Engl J Med.* 2009;361(14):1329–38.
- **Takeaways:**
  - CRT combined with ICD decreases mortality (0.5% absolute reduction) and risk of nonfatal heart failure events (8.1% absolute reduction; primarily HF exacerbation hospitalizations) in HFrEF (LVEF <= 30%) with wide QRS (>= 130 msec).
- **Notes:**
  - This trial is consistent with the COMPANION Trial (Bristow MR et al, *N Engl J Med* 2004).
  - CRT-D = CRT with defibrillator
  - CRT-P = CRT with pacemaker

Practice

Patients with moderate to severe mitral regurgitation are considered for MitraClip therapy due to functional mitral regurgitation's association with accelerating progression of HFrEF.

Evidence

- **Source:** COAPT Trial. Stone GW, Lindenfeld J, Abraham WT, et al. Transcatheter mitral-valve repair in patients with heart failure. *N Engl J Med.* 2018;379:2307–16.
- **Takeaways:**
  - First trial to show that MitraClip (transcatheter mitral valve repair) improves mortality beyond optimal medical therapy alone
- **Notes:**
  - This is a huge area of investigation now, both with regard to primary and functional MR.
  - Functional MR is five times as prevalent as primary MR.

HFpEF (CHRONIC MANAGEMENT)

Practice

Patients with HFpEF are often prescribed long-term MRA therapy.

Evidence

- **Source:** TOPCAT Trial. Pitt B, Pfeffer MA, Assmann SF, et al. Spironolactone for heart failure with preserved ejection fraction. *N Engl J Med.* 2014;370:1383–92.
- **Takeaways:**
  - No reduction in mortality or HF hospitalizations in patients with HFpEF
- **Source:** De Denus S, O'Meara E, Desai AS, et al. Spironolactone metabolites in TOPCAT—new insights into regional variation. *N Engl J Med.* 2017;376:1690–1692.
- **Takeaways:**
  - 18% reduction in mortality and HF hospitalizations in HFpEF patients
    - Storytime: A retrospective analysis found that the trial arms in Russia and Georgia likely withheld spironolactone from trial participants for personal gain. Isolating the North America and South America trial arms demonstrated a significant mortality benefit in patients with HFpEF.

- **Notes:**
  - Always check for normal potassium levels prior to initiation and monitor periodically for hyperkalemia.
  - Eplerenone may be used if spironolactone induces unwanted gynecomastia (per EMPHASIS-HF trial).
  - Trials investigating HFpEF always exclude the etiology of HFpEF, which is increasingly thought to be a mixed clinical syndrome.

Practice

Patients with HFpEF are routinely encouraged to partake in aerobic exercise.

Evidence

- **Source:** HF-ACTION Trial. O'Conner CM, Whellan DJ, Lee KL, et al. Efficacy and safety of exercise training in patients with chronic heart failure: HF-ACTION randomized controlled trial. *JAMA.* 2009;301(14):1439–50.
- **Takeaways:**
  - An aerobic exercise training program in conjunction with optimized medical therapy modestly improved clinical outcomes.
- **Source:** Pandey A, Parashar A, Kumbhani D, et al. Exercise training in patients with heart failure and preserved ejection fraction: meta-analysis of randomized control trials. *Circ Heart Fail.* 2015;8(1):33–40.
- **Takeaways:**
  - Significantly improved cardiorespiratory fitness and quality of life
  - No change in diastolic function
- **Notes:**
  - Aerobic exercise is currently one of the most effective therapeutic interventions for clinical outcomes in HFpEF.

HEART FAILURE EXACERBATION

Practice

NT-proBNP is a common first-line tool to exclude heart failure exacerbation.

Evidence

- **Source:** Breathing Not Properly Trial. Maisel AS, Krishnaswamy P, Nowak RM, et al. Rapid measurement of B-type natriuretic peptide in the emergency diagnosis of heart failure. *N Engl J Med.* 2002;347:161–7.
- **Takeaways:**
  - Initial trial that demonstrated BNP measurements were useful for establishing or excluding a diagnosis of HF
- **Source:** PRIDE Study. Januzzi JL, Camargo CA, Anwaruddin S, et al. The N-terminal Pro-BNP investigation of dyspnea in the emergency department (PRIDE) study. *Am J Cardiol.* 2005;95(8):948–54.
- **Takeaways:**
  - NT-proBNP cutoff for ruling out HF: <300
  - NT-proBNP cutoff for likely HF: >450 (>900 for age 50+)
- **Source:** TIME-CHF Trial. Pfisterer M, Buser P, Rickli H, et al. BNP-guided vs symptom-guided heart failure therapy: the trial of intensified vs standard medical therapy in elderly patients with congestive heart failure (TIME-CHF) randomized trial. *JAMA.* 2009;301(4):383–92.

- **Takeaways:**
  - NT-proBNP-guided HF therapy did not improve clinical outcomes or quality of life compared to symptom-guided therapy.
- **Notes:**
  - Always compare to prior baseline if possible!
  - BNP is elevated in renal failure patients and females.
  - BNP is decreased in obesity and HFpEF.
  - Age adjustments for BNP cutoffs:
    - <50: 450
    - 50 to 75: 900
    - 75+: 1800

Practice

In acute HF exacerbation, high-dose IV diuresis is administered by either bolus or drip.

Evidence

- **Source:** DOSE Trial. Felker GM, Lee KL, Bull DA, et al. Diuretic strategies in patients with acute decompensated heart failure. *N Engl J Med.* 2011;364:797–805.
- **Takeaways:**
  - No difference between intermittent bolus or continuous drip IV diuresis
  - High-dose diuresis is better than low-dose diuresis for symptomatic improvement.
- **Notes:**
  - High-dose diuresis does incur slightly more renal impairment but is deemed a reversible and acceptable tradeoff.
  - No equipoise to study diuretics versus placebo as ALL prior HFrEF/HFpEF trials are on a background of diuretic therapy

Practice

Outpatient guideline-directed medical therapy (GDMT) is generally continued during acute HF exacerbations.

Evidence

- **Source:** B-CONVINCED Trial. Jondeau G, Neuder Y, Eicher JC, et al. B-CONVINCED: Beta-blocker CONtinuation Vs. INterruption in patients with Congestive heart failure hospitalizED for a decompensation episode. *Eur Heart J.* 2009;30(18):2186–92.
- **Takeaways:**
  - Home beta-blocker regimen continuation during acute HF exacerbation neither delays nor decreases improvement.
- **Notes:**
  - Must first rule out of cardiogenic shock, bradycardia, or other contraindications

Practice

If significant pulmonary edema, early use of noninvasive positive pressure ventilation (NIPPV) may improve mortality and decrease intubation.

Evidence

- **Source:** Masip J, Roque M, Sánchez B, et al. Noninvasive ventilation in acute cardiogenic pulmonary edema: systematic review and meta-analysis. *JAMA.* 2005;294(24):3124.

- **Source:** Weng CL, Zhao YT, Liu QH, et al. Meta-analysis: noninvasive ventilation in acute cardiogenic pulmonary edema. *Ann Intern Med.* 2010;152(9):590–600.
- **Takeaways:**
  - Noninvasive ventilation reduces the need for intubation and mortality in patients with acute cardiogenic pulmonary edema.
- **Notes:**
  - A 2010 meta-analysis found that continuous positive airway pressure more significantly reduced mortality in patients with acute cardiogenic pulmonary edema secondary to myocardial ischemia/infarction.

Practice

Low-dose dopamine and/or low-dose nesiritide are ***not*** used in acute HF exacerbations to improve renal perfusion.

Evidence
- **Source:** ROSE-AHF Trial. Chen HH, Anstrom KJ, Givertz MM, et al. Low-dose dopamine or low-dose nesiritide in acute heart failure with renal dysfunction: the ROSE acute heart failure randomized trial. *JAMA.* 2013;310(23):2533–43.
- **Takeaways:**
  - Low-dose dopamine and/or nesiritide did not improve decongestion or renal function in participants with acute HF and renal dysfunction.

Practice

Ultrafiltration is an option in patients with cardiorenal syndrome or true diuresis resistance.

Evidence
- **Source:** UNLOAD Trial. Costanzo MR, Guglin ME, Saltzberg MT, et al. Ultrafiltration versus intravenous diuretics for patients hospitalized for acute decompensated heart failure. *J Am Coll Cardiol.* 2007;49(6):675–83.
- **Takeaways:**
  - In acute HF exacerbation, compared to IV diuresis, ultrafiltration safely produced greater weight and fluid loss and fewer readmissions.
  - No difference in kidney function or length of hospitalization
- **Notes:**
  - First trial comparing ultrafiltration to diuresis in acute HF exacerbation
- **Source:** CARRESS-HF. Bart BA, Goldsmith SR, Lee KL, et al. Ultrafiltration in decompensated heart failure with cardiorenal syndrome. *N Engl J Med.* 2012;367:2296–304.
- **Takeaways:**
  - In acute HF with cardiorenal syndrome, ultrafiltration is inferior to medical therapy in preserving renal function, comparable in weight loss, and associated with more adverse events.
- **Notes:**
  - Clarified the role of ultrafiltration in acute HF exacerbation complicated by cardiorenal syndrome

Practice

While not standard of practice yet, new evidence suggests that angiotensin receptor-neprilysin inhibitors (ARNIs) (sacubitril/valsartan) may be more effective at decreasing NT-proBNP compared to ACE inhibitors during ADHF.

Evidence
- **Source:** PIONEER-HF Trial. Velazquez EJ, Morrow DA, DeVore AD, et al. Angiotensin–neprilysin inhibition in acute decompensated heart failure. *N Engl J Med.* 2019;380:539–48.
- **Takeaways:**
  - 46.7% versus 25.3% decrease in NT-proBNP with ARNI versus ACEI use in ADHF
- **Notes:**
  - Decreasing NT-proBNP has prognostic significance.

Practice

The CardioMEMS device may be used to monitor hemodynamics for prevention of ADHF.

Evidence
- **Source:** CHAMPION Trial. Abraham WT, Adamson PB, Bourge RC, et al. Wireless pulmonary artery haemodynamic monitoring in chronic heart failure: a randomised controlled trial. *Lancet.* 2011;377:658–66.
- **Takeaways:**
  - Significant reduction in heart failure hospitalization when managed with CardioMEMS device
  - NYHA class III HF patients
- **Source:** Givertz MM, Stevenson LW, Costanzo MR, et al. Pulmonary artery pressure-guided management of patients with heart failure and reduced ejection fraction. *J Am Coll Cardiol.* 2017;70(15):1875–86.
- **Takeaways:**
  - CardioMEMS-guided therapy for patients on optimal GDMT can decrease mortality (32%) and hospitalization (28%).
- **Notes:**
  - CardioMEMS is a wireless pulmonary artery pressure measurement device.

Hypertension

PRACTICE

Patients with hypertension should follow a diet rich in fruits, vegetables, and low-fat dairy foods and with reduced saturated and total fat.

Evidence
- **Source:** DASH Trial. Appel LJ et al for the DASH Collaborative Research Group. A clinical trial of the effects of dietary patterns on blood pressure. *N Engl J Med.* Apr 17, 1997;336:1117–24.
- **Takeaways:**
  - Compared to the control diet (lower in DASH components and higher in fats), the DASH diet decreased BP by approximately 5.5/3.0 mm Hg.
  - Unfortunately, no cardiovascular outcomes were studied in this trial.
- **Notes:**
  - The DASH diet is the only diet with proven large-scale clinical trial evidence for improving blood pressure.

PRACTICE

Three classes (ACE inhibitors, CCBs, and thiazides) of medications may be used as first-line therapy for treatment of hypertension.

Evidence

- **Source:** ALLHAT Trial. Wright JT et al for the ALLHAT Collaborative Research Group. The Antihypertensive and Lipid-Lowering Treatment to Prevent Heart Attack Trial. Major outcomes in high-risk hypertensive patients randomized to angiotensin-converting enzyme inhibitor or calcium channel blocker vs diuretic: the Antihypertensive and Lipid-Lowering Treatment to Prevent Heart Attack Trial (ALLHAT). *JAMA.* Dec 18, 2002;288:2981–97.
- **Takeaways:**
  - ACEI, CCB, and thiazide performed approximately equally for cardiovascular mortality and nonfatal MI.
  - However, chlorthalidone decreased the incidence of HF compared to the other drugs.
  - Initially, there existed a fourth arm doxazosin—which was terminated due to early signals of significantly increased HF.
- **Notes:**
  - Compared with hydrochlorothiazide, chlorthalidone has a longer half-life.
  - ACE inhibitors should not be utilized as first-line therapy in African American patients due to reduced benefit and increased risk of angioedema.

PRACTICE

The combination of ACEI plus CCBs may potentially decrease cardiovascular risk compared to ACEI plus thiazide combination treatments.

Evidence

- **Source:** ACCOMPLISH Trial. Jamerson K et al. for the ACCOMPLISH Trial Investigators. Benazepril plus amlodipine or hydrochlorothiazide for hypertension in high-risk patients. *N Engl J Med.* Dec 4, 2008;359:2417–28.
- **Takeaways:**
  - The combination with CCBs demonstrated a 2.2% absolute risk reduction in cardiovascular mortality and morbidity.
- **Notes:**
  - Compared with hydrochlorothiazide, chlorthalidone has a longer half-life.
  - Interestingly, hydrochlorothiazide is the most commonly prescribed diuretic agent for hypertension, although most studies have focused on chlorothiazide.

PRACTICE

In patients with hypertension and elevated cardiovascular risk, providers should treat to a systolic blood pressure goal of 120 mm Hg.

Evidence

- **Source:** SPRINT Trial. The SPRINT Research Group. A randomized trial of intensive versus standard blood-pressure control. *N Engl J Med.* Nov 26, 2015;373:2103–16.
- **Takeaways:**
  - Patients at increased cardiovascular risk who had their blood pressure strictly controlled to <120 mm Hg had reduced cardiovascular events and improved mortality compared to the arm with more lenient BP therapy.
  - The benefit in the intensive control arm was primarily driven by a decrease in new-onset HF or related hospitalizations.

- Slightly increased adverse events such as AKI and hypotension in the intensive control arm
- **Notes:**
  - This trial included a back-prescribing feature where patients in the lenient arm who were on antihypertensives with blood pressures under the lenient goal had their antihypertensives deprescribed or doses reduced.

PRACTICE

While there is no accepted time for taking antihypertensive medications, more evidence suggests that it may be beneficial to take at least one antihypertensive medication at nighttime.

Evidence

- **Source:** Hygia Chronotherapy Study. Hermida RC et al for the Hygia Project Investigators. Bedtime hypertension treatment improves cardiovascular risk reduction: the Hygia Chronotherapy Trial. *Eur Heart J.* Dec 21, 2020; 41(48):4565–76.
- **Takeaways:**
  - Prescription of at least one antihypertensive at bedtime improved ambulatory blood pressure control as well as reduced cardiovascular events by over 40% compared to patients taking their antihypertensives upon awakening.
- **Notes:**
  - The dipper effect in blood pressure overnight is mitigated by chronic kidney disease (CKD) and may constitute a significant reason for increased cardiovascular risk in CKD.
  - Notably, this study was conducted using ambulatory blood pressure monitoring, which is thought to be more reflective of a patient's true blood pressures.

Valvular Disease

PRACTICE

Transcatheter aortic valve replacement (TAVR) is a suitable alternative, and potentially superior, to a surgical aortic valve replacement (SAVR) in low-risk surgical patients.

Evidence

- **Source:** PARTNER A Trial. Smith CR et al for the PARTNER A Investigators. Transcatheter versus surgical aortic-valve replacement in high-risk patients. *N Engl J Med.* June 9, 2011;364:2187–98.
- **Takeaways:**
  - No difference in all-cause 1-year mortality between TAVR and SAVR in high-risk surgical candidates
  - A 5-year follow-up on the PARTNER A cohort demonstrated continued non-difference in mortality.
- **Notes:**
  - Aortic regurgitation is a potential complication of TAVR, which is somewhat dependent on the type of valve replacement utilized (i.e., is there a skirt to prevent paravalvular regurgitation?).

PRACTICE

TAVR is a suitable alternative to a SAVR in intermediate-risk surgical patients.

Evidence

- **Source:** PARTNER 2 Trial. Leon MB et al for the PARTNER 2 Investigators. Transcatheter or surgical aortic-valve replacement in intermediate-risk patients. *N Engl J Med.* Apr 28, 2016;374:1609–20.
- **Takeaways:**
  - TAVR noninferior to SAVR in death or stroke
  - TAVR had significantly lower rates of major bleeding and new onset atrial fibrillation.

PRACTICE

TAVR is a suitable alternative, and potentially superior, to a SAVR in low-risk surgical patients.

Evidence

- **Source:** PARTNER 3 Trial. Mack MJ et al for the PARTNER 3 Investigators. Transcatheter aortic-valve replacement with a balloon-expandable valve in low-risk patients. *N Engl J Med.* May 2, 2019;380(18):1695–705.
- **Takeaways:**
  - TAVR outperformed SAVR in death, rehospitalization at 1 year, or stroke.
  - 1.5% absolute reduction in death

PRACTICE

Patients with moderate to severe mitral regurgitation are considered for MitraClip therapy due to functional mitral regurgitation's association with accelerating progression of HFrEF.

Evidence

- **Source:** COAPT Trial. Stone GW, Lindenfeld J, Abraham WT, et al. Transcatheter mitral-valve repair in patients with heart failure. *N Engl J Med.* 2018;379:2307–16.
- **Takeaways:**
  - First trial to show that MitraClip (transcatheter mitral valve repair) improves mortality beyond optimal medical therapy alone
- **Notes:**
  - This is a huge area of investigation now, both with regard to primary and functional MR.
  - Functional MR is 5 times as prevalent as primary MR.

Pulmonology

Pulmonology is a specialty well-versed in multicenter clinical trials, especially in regard to critical care. This chapter selects some of the more important studies upon which current practice guidelines are based.

Acute Respiratory Distress Syndrome

PRACTICE

Neuromuscular blockade can be administered for desirable effects such as improved oxygenation; however, this is at the risk of prolonged neuromuscular weakness.

Evidence

- **Source:** Papazian L, Forel JM, Gacouin A, et al. Neuromuscular blockers in early acute respiratory distress syndrome. *N Engl J Med.* 2010 Sep 16;363(12):1107–16.
- **Source:** Moss M, Huang DT, Brower RG, et al. Early neuromuscular blockade in the acute respiratory distress syndrome. *N Engl J Med.* 2019 May 23;380(21):1997–2008.
- **Takeaways:**
  - In the 2010 trial, early administration of a neuromuscular blocking agent improved the adjusted 90-day survival and increased the time off the ventilator. However, the ROSE trial performed most recently showed no significant difference in mortality at 90 days between patients who received early and continuous paralytic agents versus those treated with lighter sedation targets.
- **Notes:**
  - Given conflicting data, routine paralysis should be refrained unless there are other indications such as ventilator desynchrony.

PRACTICE

Prone positioning of the patient improves oxygenation in the majority of patients with ARDS.

Evidence

- **Source:** Sud S, Friedrich JO, Taccone P, et al. Prone ventilation reduces mortality in patients with acute respiratory failure and severe hypoxemia: systematic review and meta-analysis. *Intensive Care Med.* 2010 Apr;36(4):585–99.

- **Source:** Guérin C, Reignier J, Richard JC, et al. Prone positioning in severe acute respiratory distress syndrome. *N Engl J Med.* 2013 Jun 6;368(23):2159–68.
- **Takeaways:**
  - Early application of prolonged prone-positioning significantly decreased 28-day and 90-day mortality compared with patients who were placed in supine position. Oxygenation improved by 27% to 39% over the first 3 days of therapy.
- **Notes:**
  - Physiologic benefits include improved lung perfusion, reduced lung compression, and reducing ventral-dorsal transpulmonary pressure difference.

PRACTICE

Low tidal volume ventilation is used to maintain O_2 while preventing ventilator induced lung injury.

Evidence

- **Source:** Brower RG, Matthay MA, Morris A, et al. Ventilation with lower tidal volumes as compared with traditional tidal volumes for acute lung injury and the acute respiratory distress syndrome. *N Engl J Med.* 2000 May 4;342(18):1301–8.
- **Takeaways:**
  - Low tidal volume ventilation decreases mortality (31% vs. 40%) and increases ventilator-free days versus higher tidal volume ventilation.
- **Notes:**
  - Initial tidal volume should be less than or equal to 6 mL/kg ideal body weight.

PRACTICE

In ARDS, conservative fluid management is superior to liberal fluid management.

Evidence

- **Source:** Wiedemann HP, Wheeler AP, Bernard GR, et al. Comparison of two fluid-management strategies in acute lung injury. *N Engl J Med.* 2006 Jun 15;354(24):2564–75.
- **Takeaways:**
  - Conservative fluid management targeting central venous pressure less than 4 mm Hg improves lung function, decreases ventilator days, and reduces ICU days compared with a liberal strategy.

PRACTICE

Dexamethasone is given to COVID-19 patients who require supplemental oxygen or invasive mechanical ventilation.

Evidence

- **Source:** RECOVERY Trial. The RECOVERY Collaborative Group. Dexamethasone in Hospitalized Patients with Covid-19. *NE Engl J Med.* 2021; 384:693–704.
- **Takeaways:**
  - Dexamethasone use in patients requiring supplemental oxygen or invasive mechanical ventilation led to improved 28-day mortality (2.8% absolute reduction).
  - Importantly, the trial also studied the use of hydroxychloroquine in COVID-19 given (potentially false) reports and found no benefit, putting an end to the debate.

- **Notes:**
  - Patients who do not require supplemental oxygen should NOT be given dexamethasone. In the RECOVERY trial, there was a hint towards worse outcomes/mortality when dexamethasone was given to patients without need for oxygen.

Asthma

PRACTICE

Patients not responding to bronchodilator therapy should receive glucocorticosteroids.

Evidence

- **Source:** Fanta CH, Rossing TH, McFadden ER Jr. Glucocorticoids in acute asthma. A critical controlled trial. *Am J Med.* 1983 May;74(5):845–51.
- **Takeaways:**
  - Corticosteroids speed the recovery of asthma patients who are unresponsive to bronchodilation therapy.

PRACTICE

Intravenous (IV) glucocorticoid therapy is not superior to PO (oral) therapy.

Evidence

- **Source:** Ratto D, Alfaro C, Sipsey J, et al. Are intravenous corticosteroids required in status asthmaticus? *JAMA.* 1988 Jul 22–29;260(4):527–9.
- **Takeaways:**
  - Between PO and IV equivalent doses of methylprednisone, there were no significant differences in the incidence of respiratory failure, forced expiratory volume, days of hospitalization, or rate of improvement in pulmonary function.
- **Notes:**
  - IV glucocorticoid steroids should be given to patients who present with impending respiratory arrest and should be transitioned to oral once they can tolerate oral administration.

PRACTICE

IV magnesium sulfate can be given to patients with asthma during a severe exacerbation not responding to initial therapy.

Evidence

- **Source:** Kew KM, Kirtchuk L, Michell CI. Intravenous magnesium sulfate for treating adults with acute asthma in the emergency department. *Cochrane Database Syst Rev.* 2014 May 28;(5):CD010909.
- **Takeaways:**
  - A single infusion of 1.2 g or 2 g IV $MgSO_4$ over 15 to 30 minutes reduces hospital admissions and improves lung function in adults with acute asthma who have not responded sufficiently to oxygen, nebulized short-acting β2-agonists, and IV corticosteroids.
- **Notes:**
  - Inhaled magnesium is of marginal benefit.
  - IV magnesium is contraindicated in the presence of renal insufficiency, and hypermagnesemia can result in muscle weakness.

PRACTICE

Long-acting beta-agonists (LABAs) should not be used as monotherapy.

Evidence

- **Source:** Nelson HS, Weiss ST, Bleecker ER, et al. The Salmeterol Multicenter Asthma Research Trial: a comparison of usual pharmacotherapy for asthma or usual pharmacotherapy plus salmeterol. *Chest.* 2006 Jan;129(1):15–26.
- **Source:** Chowdhury BA, Dal Pan G. The FDA and safe use of long-acting beta-agonists in the treatment of asthma. *N Engl J Med.* 2010 Apr 1;362(13):1169–71.
- **Takeaways:**
  - Over the course of 28 weeks, there were 8 more asthma-related deaths per 10,000 patients among patients treated with salmeterol than among those given placebo.
  - Per US Food and Drug Administration (FDA) review, the benefits of LABAs continue to outweigh the risks when used appropriately, but they should be reserved for patients whose asthma cannot be adequately managed with inhaled corticosteroids.

Bronchiectasis/Cystic Fibrosis

PRACTICE

Dual *Pseudomonas* coverage.

Evidence

- **Source:** Bilton D, Henig N, Morrissey B, Gotfried M. Addition of inhaled tobramycin to ciprofloxacin for acute exacerbations of *Pseudomonas* aeruginosa infection in adult bronchiectasis. *Chest.* 2006 Nov;130(5):1503–10.
- **Takeaways:**
  - The addition of an inhaled tobramycin solution to therapy with oral ciprofloxacin for the treatment of acute exacerbations of bronchiectasis due to *Pseudomonas aeruginosa* improved microbiologic outcome and was concordant with clinical outcome.
- **Notes:**
  - Duration of therapy currently is not well defined. Clinical experience favors 10 to 14 days of treatment.

Chronic Obstructive Pulmonary Disease

PRACTICE

In patients with moderate-to-very-severe COPD, long-acting anticholinergic agents should be the initial long-acting bronchodilator used.

Evidence

- **Source:** Vogelmeier C, Hederer B, Glaab T, et al. Tiotropium versus salmeterol for the prevention of exacerbations of COPD. *N Engl J Med.* 2011 Mar 24;364(12):1093–103.
- **Takeaways:**
  - Tiotropium increased time to first exacerbation and reduced the annual number of moderate/severe exacerbations.
- **Notes:**
  - Both long-acting muscarinic antagonists and LABAs improve quality of life.

PRACTICE

During an acute COPD exacerbation, supplemental oxygen should be titrated to pulse oxygen saturation of 88% to 92% or an arterial oxygen tension of 60 to 70 mm Hg.

Evidence

- **Source:** Austin MA, Wills KE, Blizzard L, et al. Effect of high flow oxygen on mortality in chronic obstructive pulmonary disease patients in prehospital setting: randomised controlled trial. *BMJ.* 2010 Oct 18;341:c5462.
- **Takeaways:**
  - Supplemental oxygen to SpO2 88% to 92% resulted in a lower mortality, hypercapnia, and respiratory acidosis compared with patients who received untitrated high-flow oxygen.
- **Notes:**
  - A high FiO2 is not required to correct hypoxemia in most exacerbation cases and should prompt consideration for other etiologies.

PRACTICE

For patients not requiring ICU admission, prednisone 40 mg for 5 days is sufficient for an acute COPD exacerbation.

Evidence

- **Source:** Niewoehner DE, Erbland ML, Deupree RH, et al. Effect of systemic glucocorticoids on exacerbations of chronic obstructive pulmonary disease. Department of Veterans Affairs Cooperative Study Group. *N Engl J Med.* 1999 Jun 24;340(25):1941–7.
- **Source:** Leuppi JD, Schuetz P, Bingisser R, et al. Short-term vs conventional glucocorticoid therapy in acute exacerbations of chronic obstructive pulmonary disease: the REDUCE randomized clinical trial. *JAMA.* 2013 Jun 5;309(21):2223–31.
- **Source:** Lindenauer PK, Pekow PS, Lahti MC, et al. Association of corticosteroid dose and route of administration with risk of treatment failure in acute exacerbation of chronic obstructive pulmonary disease. *JAMA.* 2010 Jun 16;303(23):2359–67.
- **Takeaways:**
  - SCCOPE trial showed no benefit of 2 weeks versus 8 weeks of glucocorticoid therapy.
  - REDUCE trial compared 5 versus 14 days of therapy, which showed no difference in time to next exacerbation or recovery in lung function.
  - Lindenau et al. in *JAMA* 2010 showed that low-dose steroids administered orally are not associated with worse outcomes than high-dose IV therapy.
- **Notes:**
  - At the end of the course, therapy can be discontinued rather than tapered if the patient has substantially recovered (<3 weeks of therapy is too brief to cause adrenal atrophy).

PRACTICE

Patients with moderate-severe COPD exacerbation exhibiting two of the three cardinal symptoms (increased dyspnea, increased sputum volume, or increase sputum purulence) should receive antibiotics.

Evidence

- **Source:** Anthonisen NR, Manfreda J, Warren CP, et al. Antibiotic therapy in exacerbations of chronic obstructive pulmonary disease. *Ann Intern Med.* 1987 Feb;106(2):196–204.

- **Source:** Vollenweider DJ, Frei A, Steurer-Stey CA, et al. Antibiotics for exacerbations of chronic obstructive pulmonary disease. *Cochrane Database Syst Rev.* 2018 Oct 29;10:CD010257.
- **Takeaways:**
  - Patients treated with antibiotics compared with placebo had increased success rate of improvement, decreased treatment failure rates, and improvement in peak flow.
- **Notes:**
  - Currently, there is insufficient evidence to support treatment of mild exacerbations.
  - Initial regimen should target *Haemophilus influenza, Moraxella catarrhalis,* and *Streptococcus pneumoniae.*

PRACTICE

During severe COPD exacerbations, noninvasive ventilation should be considered prior to invasive ventilation.

Evidence

- **Source:** Brochard L, Mancebo J, Wysocki M, et al. Noninvasive ventilation for acute exacerbations of chronic obstructive pulmonary disease. *N Engl J Med.* 1995 Sep 28;333(13):817–22.
- **Source:** Lindenauer PK, Stefan MS, Shieh MS, et al. Outcomes associated with invasive and noninvasive ventilation among patients hospitalized with exacerbations of chronic obstructive pulmonary disease. *JAMA Intern Med.* 2014 Dec;174(12):1982–93.
- **Takeaways:**
  - NIPPV trial: COPD treated with NIPPV at the time of hospitalization had lower inpatient mortality and shorter length of stay compared with traditional therapies. There are lower costs compared with those treated with invasive mechanical ventilation.
- **Notes:**
  - NPPV should be considered early in the course of respiratory failure and before severe acidosis ensues, as a means of reducing the likelihood of endotracheal intubation, treatment failure, and mortality.
  - Physiologic benefits from NIV include decreased respiratory rate, increase tidal volume, and increase minute ventilation.

PRACTICE

Smoking cessation interventions should be part of the discharge plan in every patient with COPD.

Evidence

- **Source:** Anthonisen NR, Skeans MA, Wise RA, et al. The effects of a smoking cessation intervention on 14.5-year mortality: a randomized clinical trial. Ann Intern Med. 2005 Feb 15;142(4):233–9.
- **Takeaways:**
  - All-cause mortality was significantly lower in the special intervention group compared with usual care participants.

PRACTICE

Home oxygen is prescribed for patients with COPD.

Evidence

- **Source:** Continuous or nocturnal oxygen therapy in hypoxemic chronic obstructive lung disease: a clinical trial. Nocturnal Oxygen Therapy Trial Group. *Ann Intern Med.* 1980 Sep;93(3):391–8.
- **Source:** Long term domiciliary oxygen therapy in chronic hypoxic cor pulmonale complicating chronic bronchitis and emphysema. Report of the Medical Research Council Working Party. *Lancet.* 1981 Mar 28;1(8222):681–6.
- **Takeaways:**
  - Both these trials demonstrated improved survival among patients that use oxygen long-term.

Interstitial Lung Disease

PRACTICE

Nintedanib appears to slow disease progression in idiopathic pulmonary fibrosis.

Evidence

- **Source:** Richeldi L, Costabel U, Selman M, et al. Efficacy of a tyrosine kinase inhibitor in idiopathic pulmonary fibrosis. *N Engl J Med.* 2011 Sep 22;365(12):1079–87.
- **Source:** Richeldi L, du Bois RM, Raghu G, et al. Efficacy and safety of nintedanib in idiopathic pulmonary fibrosis. *N Engl J Med.* 2014 May 29;370(22):2071–82.
- **Takeaways:**
  - Nintedanib reduced the decline in lung function, resulted in fewer exacerbations, and preserved quality of life.

PRACTICE

It is recommended against using azathioprine/prednisone/N-acetylcysteine (NAC) together in patients with ILD.

Evidence

- **Source:** Oldham JM, Ma SF, Martinez FJ, et al. TOLLIP, MUC5B, and the response to N-acetylcysteine among individuals with idiopathic pulmonary fibrosis. *Am J Respir Crit Care Med.* 2015 Dec 15;192(12):1475–82.
- **Notes:**
  - Sometimes NAC monotherapy is given because of its minimal side effects, but there is no benefit seen in some randomized controlled trials.

Obstructive Sleep Apnea

PRACTICE

Continuous positive airway pressure remains the mainstay of therapy for adults with OSA.

Evidence

- **Source:** Jonas DE, Amick HR, Feltner C, et al. Screening for obstructive sleep apnea in adults: evidence report and systematic review for the US Preventive Services Task Force. *JAMA.* 2017 Jan 24;317(4):415–33.
- **Takeaways:**
  - CPAP significantly reduces the apnea-hypopnea index (difference of −33.8 events/per), improves daytime sleepiness, and reduces both systolic/diastolic blood pressure.

- **Notes:**
  - No appreciable effect on mortality has been reported.

Pulmonary Arterial Hypertension

PRACTICE

Endothelial receptor antagonists are first-line therapies in PAH.

Evidence

- **Source:** Pulido T, Adzerikho I, Channick RN, et al. Macitentan and morbidity and mortality in pulmonary arterial hypertension. *N Engl J Med.* 2013 Aug 29;369(9):809–18.
- **Takeaways:**
  - Macitentan significantly reduced morbidity and mortality versus placebo. The primary end point in this study was time from initiation of treatment to the first occurrence of a composite end point of death, atrial septostomy, lung transplant, or worsening of pulmonary arterial hypertension.

PRACTICE

Phosphodiesterase-5 (PDE-5) inhibitors improve quality of life in patients with PAH.

Evidence

- **Source:** Galiè N, Ghofrani HA, Torbicki A, et al. Sildenafil citrate therapy for pulmonary arterial hypertension. *N Engl J Med.* 2005 Nov 17;353(20):2148–57.
- **Takeaways:**
  - Sildenafil in this study improved exercise capacity, World Health Organization (WHO) functional class, and hemodynamics compared with placebo.

Gastroenterology

Alcoholic Hepatitis

PRACTICE

In patients with severe alcoholic hepatitis, 40 mg of prednisolone is given for 28 days with a 16-day taper if the patient responds.

Evidence

- **Source:** Pavlov CS, Varganova DL, Casazza G, et al. Glucocorticosteroids for people with alcoholic hepatitis. *Cochrane Database Syst Rev.* 2019 Apr 9;4:CD001511.
- **Source:** Ramond MJ, Poynard T, Rueff B, et al. A randomized trial of prednisolone in patients with severe alcoholic hepatitis. *N Engl J Med.* 1992 Feb 20;326(8):507–12.
- **Takeaways:**
  - Sixteen of 29 placebo recipients had died compared with 4 of 32 prednisolone recipients, thus suggesting that treatment of prednisolone improved the short-term survival of patients with severe biopsy-proven alcoholic hepatitis.
- **Notes:**
  - Prednisolone is given instead of prednisone because the latter requires conversion in the liver. Some authorities recommend using pentoxifylline instead given conflicting results with steroids.

PRACTICE

Pentoxifylline is given 400 mg three times per day as an alternative to glucocorticoids for the treatment of severe alcoholic hepatitis.

Evidence

- **Source:** Akriviadis E, Botla R, Briggs W, et al. Pentoxifylline improves short-term survival in severe acute alcoholic hepatitis: a double-blind, placebo-controlled trial. *Gastroenterology.* 2000 Dec;119(6):1637–48.

- **Source:** Singh S, Murad MH, Chandar AK, et al. Comparative effectiveness of pharmacological interventions for severe alcoholic hepatitis: a systematic review and network meta-analysis. *Gastroenterology.* 2015 Oct;149(4):958–970.e12.
- **Takeaways:**
  - In the initial 2000 study, 24.5% of patients who received pentoxifylline compared with 46.1% of patients who received placebo died during the index hospitalization, with the benefit appearing to be related to a significant decrease in the development of hepatorenal syndrome (HRS).
  - In the network meta-analysis, low-quality evidence demonstrated that pentoxifylline decreased short-term mortality.
- **Notes:**
  - Use of pentoxifylline remains controversial because other studies and meta-analyses have failed to show a benefit with regard to mortality.

PRACTICE

In patients with severe alcoholic hepatitis, some practitioners use combination therapy of prednisolone + N-acetylcysteine.

Evidence

- **Source:** Nguyen-Khac E, Thevenot T, Piquet MA, et al. Glucocorticoids plus N-acetylcysteine in severe alcoholic hepatitis. *N Engl J Med.* 2011 Nov 10;365(19):1781–9.
- **Takeaways:**
  - In this study, 85 out of 174 patients received combination therapy versus 89 who received only prednisolone. Mortality was significantly lower at 1 month in the combination group compared with the prednisolone-only group (8% vs. 24%); however, it was not at 3 or 6 months.
- **Notes:**
  - Death secondary to HRS was also seen less in the combination therapy group.

PRACTICE

Prednisolone is sometimes, at provider discretion, given to patients with alcoholic hepatitis.

Evidence

- **Source:** STOPAH Trial. Thursz MR, Richardson P, Allison M, et al.; STOPAH Trial. Prednisolone or pentoxifylline for alcoholic hepatitis. *N Engl J Med.* 2015;372:1619–28.
- **Takeaways:**
  - Prednisolone led to a trend (odds ratio [OR] 0.72, $P = .06$) toward reduced 28-day mortality but had no associated improvement in outcomes at 3 months or 1 year.
  - Pentoxifylline was not associated with a mortality benefit in patients with alcoholic hepatitis.

Acute Liver Failure

PRACTICE

A short course of N-acetylcysteine (72 hours) is given in early stages of liver failure to patients who are not candidates for liver transplantation and to patients with an indeterminate cause for acute liver failure.

Evidence

- **Source**: Lee WM, Hynan LS, Rossaro L, et al. Intravenous N-acetylcysteine improves transplant-free survival in early stage non-acetaminophen acute liver failure. *Gastroenterology.* 2009 Sep;137(3):856–64, 864.e1.
- **Takeaways:**
  - A placebo-controlled trial involving 173 patients with acute liver failure due to causes other than acetaminophen found significantly high transplant-free survival (40% vs. 27%).
- **Notes:**
  - Benefit of N-acetylcysteine appears to be confined to patients with early-stage hepatic encephalopathy.

Ascites/Cirrhosis

PRACTICE

Serum-ascites albumin gradient (SAAG) is used in order to determine the cause of ascites formation.

Evidence

- **Source:** Runyon BA, Montano AA, Akriviadis EA, et al. The serum-ascites albumin gradient is superior to the exudate-transudate concept in the differential diagnosis of ascites. *Ann Intern Med.* 1992 Aug 1;117(3):215–20.
- **Takeaways:**
  - The SAAG correctly differentiated causes of ascites due to portal hypertension from those that were not due to portal hypertension 96.7% of the time compared with the old exudate-transudate concept (55.6% of the time).
- **Notes:**
  - A high gradient (1.1 g/dL) indicates the ascites is due to hypertension with 97% accuracy.

PRACTICE

In patients undergoing large-volume paracentesis, intravenous (IV) albumin is given to avoid renal and electrolyte complications.

Evidence

- **Source:** Ginès P, Titó L, Arroyo V, et al. Randomized comparative study of therapeutic paracentesis with and without intravenous albumin in cirrhosis. *Gastroenterology.* 1988 Jun;94(6):1493–502.
- **Takeaways:**
  - A total of 105 patients were randomly allocated into two groups (52 received IV albumin + large-volume paracentesis versus 53 patients who only underwent large-volume paracentesis).
  - The patients who did not receive IV albumin had significant increases in blood urea nitrogen (BUN), marked elevation in plasma renin activity and aldosterone, and a significant reduction in serum sodium concentration.
- **Notes:**
  - It is suggested to give 12.5 g of albumin for every 2 L in excess of 5 L paracentesis.

PRACTICE

A transjugular intrahepatic portosystemic shunt (TIPS) procedure can be performed in selected patients who have diuretic-resistant ascites.

Evidence

- **Source:** Rössle M, Ochs A, Gülberg V, et al. A comparison of paracentesis and transjugular intrahepatic portosystemic shunting in patients with ascites. *N Engl J Med.* 2000 Jun 8;342(23):1701–7.
- **Takeaways:**
  - In comparison with large-volume paracentesis, the creation of a TIPS improves the chance of survival without liver transplantations in patients with refractory or recurrent ascites.
  - The probability of survival without lower transplantation was 69% at 1 year and 58% at 2 years in the shunt group versus 52% and 32%, respectively, in the paracentesis group.
- **Notes:**
  - Patients who are not good candidates for TIPS include those with high Model for End-Stage Liver Disease (MELD) scores (>18), who have heart failure, or who have a Child-Pugh class C cirrhosis.

PRACTICE

In patients with spontaneous bacterial peritonitis (SBP) with renal dysfunction, IV albumin is used in conjunction with antibiotics in patients.

Evidence

- **Source:** Sort P, Navasa M, Arroyo V, et al. Effect of intravenous albumin on renal impairment and mortality in patients with cirrhosis and spontaneous bacterial peritonitis. *N Engl J Med.* 1999 Aug 5;341(6):403–9.
- **Takeaways:**
  - A total of 126 patients with cirrhosis and SBP were randomly assigned to be given cefotaxime (63 patients) or cefotaxime and IV albumin (63 patients). Renal impairment developed in 21 patients in the cefotaxime group (33%) versus 6 patients in the combined group.
- **Notes:**
  - Renal failure develops in 30% to 40% of patients with SBP and is a major cause of death. Albumin should be given at a rate of 1.5 g/kg body weight initially.

PRACTICE

Antibiotic prophylaxis is given to high-risk cirrhotic patients with ascites.

Evidence

- **Source:** Saab S, Hernandez JC, Chi AC, Tong MJ. Oral antibiotic prophylaxis reduces spontaneous bacterial peritonitis occurrence and improves short-term survival in cirrhosis: a meta-analysis. *Am J Gastroenterol.* 2009 Apr;104(4):993–1001; quiz 1002.
- **Takeaways:**
  - In this systematic review, eight studies with a total of 647 patients were identified and included in the analysis.

- The overall mortality rate was 16% for treated patients versus 25% for the control group. This study also demonstrated a survival benefit at 3 months.
- **Notes:**
  - High-risk features include patients who have gastrointestinal (GI) bleeding or have had one or more episodes of SBP and those with impaired renal function.

PRACTICE

Nonselective beta-blockers are used to prevent against variceal hemorrhage in patients with cirrhosis.

Evidence

- **Source:** Hayes PC, Davis JM, Lewis JA, Bouchier IA. Meta-analysis of value of propranolol in prevention of variceal haemorrhage. *Lancet*. 1990 Jul 21;336(8708):153–6.
- **Takeaways:**
  - This meta-analysis included 797 patients and found that patients treated with beta-blockers had improved outcomes compared with controls. They had lower rates of bleeding (12% vs. 23% in controls) and fewer deaths due to bleeding (5% vs. 10%).
- **Notes:**
  - The goal of pharmacologic treatment in this case is to decrease portal venous inflow. Nonselective beta-blockers accomplish this by inhibitor adrenergic mesenteric arteriole dilation, which in turn leads to unopposed alpha-adrenergic–mediated vasoconstriction and therefore a decrease in portal flow.
  - Cardioselective beta-blockers such as atenolol do not have as dramatic an effect in reducing portal venous pressure.
  - In the setting of SBP, nonselective beta-blockers should be discontinued because they are associated with worse renal outcomes, infection, and potentially increased mortality.

PRACTICE

A combination of endoscopic and drug therapy is used to stop variceal rebleeding in cirrhosis.

Evidence

- **Source:** Gonzalez R, Zamora J, Gomez-Camarero J, et al. Meta-analysis: combination endoscopic and drug therapy to prevent variceal rebleeding in cirrhosis. *Ann Intern Med*. 2008 Jul 15;149(2):109–22.
- **Takeaways:**
  - This meta-analysis included 1860 patients and found combined therapy reduced overall rebleeding more than endoscopic therapy or beta-blocker therapy alone (pooled relative risk [RR] 0.68 and 0.71, respectively). Combination therapy additionally reduced variceal rebleeding and variceal recurrence.
- **Notes:**
  - Effects in this analysis were independent of the endoscopic procedure performed. There was no effect on mortality in this study.

PRACTICE

Lactulose is used for the prevention of recurrence of hepatic encephalopathy in patients with cirrhosis.

Evidence

- **Source:** Sharma BC, Sharma P, Agrawal A, Sarin SK. Secondary prophylaxis of hepatic encephalopathy: an open-label randomized controlled trial of lactulose versus placebo. *Gastroenterology.* 2009 Sep;137(3):885–91, 891.e1.
- **Takeaways:**
  - This meta-analysis included 1860 patients and found combined therapy reduced overall rebleeding more than endoscopic therapy or beta-blocker therapy alone (pooled RR 0.68 and 0.71, respectively). Combination therapy additionally reduced variceal rebleeding and variceal recurrence.
- **Notes:**
  - Effects in this analysis were independent of the endoscopic procedure performed. There was no effect on mortality in this study.

PRACTICE

Rifaximin is used as secondary prophylaxis of hepatic encephalopathy in cirrhotic patients.

Evidence

- **Source:** Bass NM, Mullen KD, Sanyal A, et al. Rifaximin treatment in hepatic encephalopathy. *N Engl J Med.* 2010 Mar 25;362(12):1071–81.
- **Takeaways:**
  - In this randomized, double-blind, placebo-controlled trial, 299 patients who were in remission from recurrent hepatic encephalopathy were either given rifaximin (140 patients) or placebo (159 patients).
  - Rifaximin was shown to significantly reduce the risk of an episode of hepatic encephalopathy (hazard ratio 0.42) over a 6-month period. A total of 13.6% of patients in the rifaximin group had a hospitalization involving hepatic encephalopathy compared with 22.6% of patients in the placebo group.
- **Notes:**
  - More than 90% of the patients in both arms were receiving concurrent lactulose therapy as well.

PRACTICE

A combination of midodrine + octreotide + albumin is used in the treatment of type I HRS.

Evidence

- **Source:** Angeli P, Volpin R, Gerunda G, et al. Reversal of type 1 hepatorenal syndrome with the administration of midodrine and octreotide. *Hepatology.* 1999 Jun;29(6):1690–7.
- **Source:** Esrailian E, Pantangco ER, Kyulo NL, et al. Octreotide/Midodrine therapy significantly improves renal function and 30-day survival in patients with type 1 hepatorenal syndrome. *Dig Dis Sci.* 2007 Mar;52(3):742–8.
- **Takeaways:**
  - Prior to this study, patients with type I HRS were treated with nonpressor doses of dopamine and albumin.
  - In this study, 13 patients were enrolled, with 5 of them treated with midodrine, octreotide, and albumin versus 8 patients who were treated with dopamine and albumin.

- The patients who were treated with midodrine, octreotide, and albumin were shown to have an improvement renal plasma flow, glomerular filtration rate, and urinary sodium excretion.
- A follow-up study included 81 patients, 60 of whom were treated with octreotide/midodrine and 21 of whom were controls. Mortality was significantly lower in the treatment group (43%) versus the control group (71%).
- **Notes:**
  - Midodrine works as a systemic vasoconstrictor, and octreotide inhibits the release of endogenous vasodilators. Both work together to improve renal and systemic hemodynamics.

PRACTICE

The MELD score is used predict mortality among patients with chronic liver disease and is applied towards the allocation of donor livers.

Evidence

- **Source:** Wiesner R, Edwards E, Freeman R, et al. Model for end-stage liver disease (MELD) and allocation of donor livers. *Gastroenterology.* 2003 Jan;124(1):91 6.
- **Takeaways:**
  - In this study cohort, the MELD score was applied to estimate 3-month mortality to 3437 adult liver transplant candidates.
  - Patients with a MELD score less than 9 experienced a 1.9% mortality, whereas patients having a MELD score of 40 or greater had a mortality rate of 71.3%.
- **Notes:**
  - Midodrine works as a systemic vasoconstrictor, and octreotide inhibits the release of endogenous vasodilators. Both work together to improve renal and systemic hemodynamics.

PRACTICE

Ursodeoxycholic acid (UDCA) is used as first-line therapy in primary biliary cirrhosis (PBC).

Evidence

- **Source:** Lindor KD, Dickson ER, Baldus WP, et al. Ursodeoxycholic acid in the treatment of primary biliary cirrhosis. *Gastroenterology.* 1994 May;106(5):1284–90.
- **Source:** Corpechot C, Carrat F, Bahr A, et al. The effect of ursodeoxycholic acid therapy on the natural course of primary biliary cirrhosis. *Gastroenterology.* 2005 Feb;128(2):297–303.
- **Takeaways:**
  - A double-blind, placebo-controlled trial of UDCA was conducted in 180 patients (89 receiving UDCA and 91 placebo) with PBC to define the efficacy and safety of UDCA.
  - Patients who received UDCA had significantly delayed treatment failure compared with the placebo group. In the 2005 study, 262 patients with PBC were treated with UDCA to assess its effect on the natural course of PBC.
  - It was shown that the survival rates of patients in stage 1 and stage 2 PBC were similar to that in the control population (relative 0.8), whereas the probability of death remained increased in treated patients with later histologic stages (RR 2.2).
- **Notes:**
  - The extent of the biochemical response to UDCA during the first year of therapy is a simple and useful marker of long-term prognosis.

PRACTICE

Liver transplant is a consideration (using the Milan Criteria) for cirrhotic patients with hepato-cellular carcinoma.

Evidence

- **Source:** Mazzaferro V, Regalia E, Doci R, et al. Liver transplantation for the treatment of small hepatocellular carcinomas in patients with cirrhosis. *N Engl J Med.* 1996;334:693–700.
- **Takeaways:**
  - Prospective study on the role of liver transplant in cirrhotic patients with hepatocellular carcinoma
  - Liver transplant associated with improved mortality and outcomes up to 5 years
  - Milan Criteria derived from the careful patient selection in this study
    - Single lesion less than 5 cm or maximum 3 lesions less than 3 cm
    - No extrahepatic manifestations
    - No evidence of gross vascular invasion

Cholecystitis/Cholelithiasis

PRACTICE

Statins are used post cholecystectomy to decrease risk of gallstones.

Evidence

- **Source:** Bodmer M, Brauchli YB, Krähenbühl S, et al. Statin use and risk of gallstone disease followed by cholecystectomy. *JAMA.* 2009 Nov 11;302(18):2001–7.
- **Takeaways:**
  - In this case-control analysis, a total of 27,035 patients with cholecystectomy and 106,531 matched controls were identified, including 2396 patients and 8868 controls who had statin use. The adjusted ORs for current use of statins (20 or more prescriptions within the last 90 days) were 0.6 across age, sex, and body mass index categories. Thus it suggested that long-term use of statins was associated with a decreased risk of gallstones post cholecystectomy.
- **Notes:**
  - Statins reduce biliary cholesterol secretion, and long-term use is associated with a reduction in gallbladder disease. However, the efficacy of statins in gallstone dissolution has not been demonstrated.

PRACTICE

Patients with acute cholecystitis, who are surgical candidates, should undergo cholecystectomy as soon as seemingly possible.

Evidence

- **Source:** Gutt CN, Encke J, Köninger J, et al. Acute cholecystitis: early versus delayed cholecystectomy, a multicenter randomized trial (ACDC study, NCT00447304). *Ann Surg.* 2013 Sep;258(3):385–93.
- **Source:** Gurusamy K, Samraj K, Gluud C, et al. Meta-analysis of randomized controlled trials on the safety and effectiveness of early versus delayed laparoscopic cholecystectomy for acute cholecystitis. *Br J Surg.* 2010 Feb;97(2):141–50.

- **Takeaways:**
  - In these studies, early laparoscopic cholecystectomy resulted in a shorter total hospital stay (4 days) compared with delayed surgery. In the 2013 study, the morbidity rate was significantly lower in the early surgery group (11.8%) compared with the delayed surgery group (34.4%).
- **Notes:**
  - Contraindications to laparoscopic cholecystectomy are primarily related to anesthetic concerns and include diffuse peritonitis with hemodynamic compromise and uncontrolled bleeding disorders.

Gastrointestinal Bleeding/Peptic Ulcer Disease

PRACTICE

IV erythromycin can be given before endoscopy to improve stomach cleansing and quality of endoscopic examination in patients with an upper GI bleed.

Evidence

- **Source:** Carbonell N, Pauwels A, Serfaty L, et al. Erythromycin infusion prior to endoscopy for acute upper gastrointestinal bleeding: a randomized, controlled, double-blind trial. *Am J Gastroenterol.* 2006 Jun;101(6):1211–5.
- **Takeaways:**
  - In this double-blind study, 100 patients admitted for upper GI bleeding were randomly assigned to receive either gastric lavage + IV erythromycin or gastric lavage plus placebo. The endoscopist was able to entirely visualize the gastric mucosa of 65% of patients in the erythromycin group versus 44% in the placebo group.
  - Clots were found in the stomach in 30% of the erythromycin group versus 52% in the placebo group.
- **Notes:**
  - Erythromycin promotes gastric emptying based upon its ability to be an agonist of motilin receptors.
  - As of the 2019 guidelines, this is not routinely recommended, although it is still a viable option in certain cases.

PRACTICE

Patients with cirrhosis who present with upper GI bleeding are given prophylactic antibiotics, preferably before endoscopy.

Evidence

- **Source:** Fernández J, Ruiz del Arbol L, Gómez C, et al. Norfloxacin vs ceftriaxone in the prophylaxis of infections in patients with advanced cirrhosis and hemorrhage. *Gastroenterology.* 2006 Oct;131(4):1049–56.
- **Takeaways:**
  - Twelve trials (1241 patients) evaluating antibiotic prophylaxis against placebo were included in this study. Prophylaxis was associated with reduced mortality (RR of 0.79), mortality from bacterial infections (RR 0.43), bacterial infections (RR 0.35), rebleeding (RR 0.53), and days of hospitalization.
- **Notes:**
  - Ceftriaxone is typically used because most infections are due to gram-negative bacteria.

- There are a number of meta-analyses that support these outcomes. The aforementioned trial is one of the key trials, although this practice is not based on a single landmark trial.

PRACTICE

Famotidine or proton pump inhibitors (PPIs) are given to patients who take aspirin to prevent ulcers.

Evidence

- **Source:** Taha AS, McCloskey C, Prasad R, Bezlyak V. Famotidine for the prevention of peptic ulcers and esophagitis in patients taking low-dose aspirin (FAMOUS): a phase III, randomised, double-blind, placebo-controlled trial. *Lancet.* 2009 Jul 11;374(9684):119–25.
- **Takeaways:**
  - In this randomized, double-blind study, patients were assigned to receive famotidine versus placebo; 3.4% of the patients in the famotidine group were found to have gastric ulcers compared with the 15% of patients in the placebo arm. In addition, duodenal ulcers were seen in 0.5% of patients in the famotidine arm versus 8.5% of patients in the placebo arm. Lastly, erosive esophagitis was seen in 4.4% of patients in the famotidine group versus 19.0% of patients in the placebo group.

PRACTICE

After endoscopic treatment of bleeding peptic ulcers, high-dose infusion of PPIs is used to reduce the risk of recurrent bleeding.

Evidence

- **Source:** Lau JY, Sung JJ, Lee KK, et al. Effect of intravenous omeprazole on recurrent bleeding after endoscopic treatment of bleeding peptic ulcers. *N Engl J Med.* 2000 Aug;343:310–316.
- **Takeaways:**
  - In this double-blind trial, patients were given either omeprazole given as a bolus IV injection followed by an infusion for 72 hours versus placebo after hemostasis had been achieved via endoscopic treatment. Bleeding recurred within 30 days in 6.7% of the patients in the omeprazole group versus 22.5% in the placebo arm. Most of the episodes of recurrent bleeding occurred during the first 3 days post endoscopic treatment.
- **Notes:**
  - All PPIs are equally effective in equipotent dosages.

PRACTICE

During an acute upper GI bleed, packed red blood cell transfusion should be given when the hemoglobin level decreases to less than 7 g/dL.

Evidence

- **Source:** Villanueva C, Colomo A, Bosch A, et al. Transfusion strategies for acute upper gastrointestinal bleeding. *N Engl J Med.* 2013 Jan 3;368(1):11–21.
- **Takeaways:**
  - A total of 225 patients were assigned to the restrictive strategy (threshold <7 g/dL) versus the more liberal strategy (threshold <9 g/dL).

- The probability of survival at 6 weeks was higher in the restrictive-strategy group (95% vs. 91%). Further bleeding occurred in 10% of the patients in the restrictive group compared with 16% in the liberal group. In addition, there were fewer complications (40% vs. 48%) in the restrictive strategy group.
- **Notes:**
  - Traditionally, the optimal transfusion threshold in the setting of acute coronary syndromes is greater than 8 g/dL. This threshold (Hb >8) also applies to asymptomatic medical patients with stable coronary artery disease.
  - The 2019 guidelines in *Annals of Internal Medicine* advocate for a transfusion threshold of 8 g/dL for everyone and higher for cardiac patients, but this has not been widely adopted yet.

Inflammatory Bowel Disease

PRACTICE

Infliximab is used in the treatment of moderate-severe Crohn disease.

Evidence

- **Source:** Hanauer SB, Feagan BG, Lichtenstein GR, et al.; ACCENT I Study Group. Maintenance infliximab for Crohn's disease: the ACCENT I randomised trial. *Lancet.* 2002;359(9317):1541–9.
- **Source:** Colombel JF, Sandborn WJ, Reinisch W, et al. Infliximab, azathioprine, or combination therapy for Crohn's disease. *N Engl J Med.* 2010 Apr 15;362(15):1383–95.
- **Takeaways:**
  - ACCENT 1 trial: Infliximab use (every 8 weeks) was associated with increased remission from Crohn disease and discontinued steroid use. This study opened the doors to investigating the role of immunomodulatory drugs such as infliximab in inflammatory bowel disease.
  - The Study of Biologic and Immunomodulator Naïve Patients in Crohn's Disease (SONIC) trial: In this randomized, double-blind trial, patients were randomly assigned to receive IV infusion of infliximab + placebo pills, azathioprine pills + IV placebo, or a combination of IV infliximab and azathioprine pills; 56.8% of patients in the combination group achieved corticosteroid-free clinical remission at 26 weeks compared with 44.4% receiving infliximab alone or 30.0% receiving azathioprine alone.
- **Notes:**
  - Key adverse side effects of infliximab (really, all biologics) include reactivation of chronic hepatitis B and latent tuberculosis, as well as drug-induced lupus.

PRACTICE

Infliximab is used in the treatment of moderate-to-severe ulcerative colitis.

Evidence

- **Source:** Rutgeerts P, Sandborn WJ, Feagan BG, et al. Infliximab for induction and maintenance therapy for ulcerative colitis. *N Engl J Med.* 2005 Dec 8;353(23):2462–76.
- **Takeaways:**
  - Active Ulcerative Colitis Trials (ACT): In the randomized, double-blind trials, patients were treated with either placebo or infliximab (5 mg or 10 mg/kg of body weight) at weeks 0, 2, 6, and every 8 weeks through week 46; 69% of patients who received 5 mg of infliximab and 61% of those who received 10 mg had a clinical response at week 8 compared with the 37% who received placebo.

- In addition, a clinical response was seen more in patients receiving infliximab at 30 weeks and 54 weeks compared with the placebo groups.
- **Notes:**
  - Prior to this trial, infliximab was established only for Crohn disease.

PRACTICE

Methotrexate is used for maintenance of remission in Crohn disease.

Evidence

- **Source:** Feagan BG, Fedorak RN, Irvine EJ, et al. A comparison of methotrexate with placebo for the maintenance of remission in Crohn's disease. North American Crohn's Study Group Investigators. *N Engl J Med.* 2000 Jun 1;342(22):1627–32.
- **Takeaways:**
  - In this double-blind, multicenter study, patients with chronically active Crohn disease who had entered remission were randomly assigned to receive a dose of 15 mg methotrexate intramuscularly once week or placebo for 40 weeks. No other treatments for Crohn disease were permitted. At week 40, 65% of patients in the methotrexate group were in remission compared with the 39% in the placebo group. Fewer patients in the methotrexate group required prednisone for relapse (28% vs. 58%).
- **Notes:**
  - Folic acid is supplemented in patients who take low-dose methotrexate.

PRACTICE

Adalimumab can be used for patients with moderate-to-severe Crohn disease who cannot tolerate infliximab.

Evidence

- **Source:** Sandborn WJ, Rutgeerts P, Enns R, et al. Adalimumab induction therapy for Crohn disease previously treated with infliximab: a randomized trial. *Ann Intern Med.* 2007 Jun 19;146(12):829–38.
- **Takeaways:**
  - Patients were randomly assigned to receive induction doses of adalimumab, 160 and 80 mg, at weeks 0 and 2, respectively, or placebo at the same time points. A total of 301 patients completed the trial; 21% of patients in the adalimumab group versus 7% of those in the placebo group achieved remission at week 4.
- **Notes:**
  - The trial did not directly compare efficacy of different anti-tumor necrosis factor agents and did not assess maintenance of response.

Nonalcoholic Fatty Liver Disease

PRACTICE

Some therapies for nonalcoholic steatohepatitis include vitamin E and pioglitazone.

Evidence

- **Source:** Sanyal AJ, Chalasani N, Kowdley KV, et al. Pioglitazone, vitamin E, or placebo for nonalcoholic steatohepatitis. *N Engl J Med.* 2010 May 6;362(18):1675–85.

- **Takeaways:**
  - In this study, patients with nonalcoholic steatohepatitis and without diabetes received pioglitazone, vitamin E, or placebo for 96 weeks. Vitamin E therapy, as compared with placebo, was associated with a significantly higher rate of improvement in nonalcoholic steatohepatitis (43% vs. 19%), but the difference in the rate of improvement with pioglitazone as compared with placebo was not significant (34% and 19%).
  - Serum alanine and aspartate aminotransferase levels were reduced with vitamin E and with pioglitazone, as compared with placebo, and both agents were associated with reductions in hepatic steatosis and lobular inflammation.
- **Notes:**
  - Vitamin E is used to reduce oxidative stress in these populations.

Pancreatitis

PRACTICE

Enteral feeding is preferred over total parenteral feeding (TPN) in patients with acute pancreatitis.

Evidence

- **Source:** Marik PE, Zaloga GP. Meta-analysis of parenteral nutrition versus enteral nutrition in patients with acute pancreatitis. *BMJ.* 2004 Jun 12;328(7453):1407.
- **Takeaways:**
  - Enteral nutrition was associated with a significantly lower incidence of infections (RR 0.45), reduced surgical interventions to control pancreatitis (RR 0.48), and a reduced length of hospital stay (mean reduction 2.9, 1.6 to 4.3 days, $P < .001$).
  - There were no significant differences in mortality between the two groups of patients.
- **Notes:**
  - Although the mechanisms by which enteral nutrition decreases infectious complications are unknown, it is thought to be related to the preservation of gut immune function and reduction of inflammation.

PRACTICE

Prophylactic antibiotics are not routinely used in the management of severe acute pancreatitis.

Evidence

- **Source:** Jafri NS, Mahid SS, Idstein SR, et al. Antibiotic prophylaxis is not protective in severe acute pancreatitis: a systematic review and meta-analysis. *Am J Surg.* 2009 Jun;197(6):806–13.
- **Takeaways:**
  - In this systemic review and meta-analysis, 502 patients were pooled from eight studies. Overall, there was no protective effect of antibiotic treatment with respect to mortality. There was no protective effect against infected necrosis or surgical intervention.
- **Notes:**
  - However, 20% of patients with acute pancreatitis may develop an extrapancreatic infection; thus antibiotics should be started while the source of the infection is being determined.

PRACTICE

The bedside index for severity in acute pancreatitis (BISAP) score is used to identify patients at risk of worsening pancreatitis.

Evidence

- **Source:** Singh VK, Wu BU, Bollen TL, et al. A prospective evaluation of the bedside index for severity in acute pancreatitis score in assessing mortality and intermediate markers of severity in acute pancreatitis. *Am J Gastroenterol.* 2009 Apr;104(4):966–71.
- **Takeaways:**
  - The BISAP score was evaluated among 397 consecutive cases of acute pancreatitis admitted at a single institution. There was a statistically significant trend for increasing mortality ($P < .0001$) with increasing BISAP score. A BISAP score of 3 or greater was associated with an increased risk of developing organ failure (OR = 7.4), persistent organ failure (OR = 12.7), and pancreatic necrosis (OR = 3.8).
- **Notes:**
  - This scoring system is easily calculated at bedside; however, it has not been validated for predicting outcomes such as length of hospital stay, need for ICU care, or need for intervention.
  - Patients are assigned 1 point for each of the following during the first 24 hours: BUN greater than 25 mg/dL, impaired mental status, presence of systemic inflammatory response syndrome, age greater than 60, or presence of a pleural effusion.

Neurology

Primary Headaches

PRACTICE

Neuroimaging is reserved for patients with headaches that demonstrate concerning histories or specific signs (e.g., elevated intracranial pressure, focal neurologic deficits).

Evidence

- **Source:** Frishberg BM. The utility of neuroimaging in the evaluation of headache in patients with normal neurologic examinations. *Neurology.* 1994;44(7):1191–7.
- **Takeaways:**
  - A total of 0.4% of computed tomography (CT) or magnetic resonance imaging (MRI) scans in patients with headaches of all types without abnormalities on neurologic exam revealed treatable lesions.
- **Notes:**
  - A complete, thorough exam is necessary in almost all neurologic patients, despite what their presumed diagnosis may be.
  - Red flags that should prompt neuroimaging in the setting of headache include:
    - Sudden onset with high severity
    - Headache with systemic signs and symptoms (fever, rash, stiff neck)
    - Focal neurologic deficits (not aura related)
    - Immunocompromise
    - Unintentional weight loss
    - Age greater than 50

PRACTICE

The POUND mnemonic is a popular tool for assessing the probability of a migraine headache.

Evidence

- **Source:** Wilson JF. In the clinic. Migraine. *Ann Intern Med.* 2007;147:(9):ITC11-1–16.

- **Takeaways:**
  - Presence of 4+ POUND symptoms has a 100% specificity for migraine
  - Presence of 3+ POUND symptoms has an 80% sensitivity for migraine
- **Notes:**
  - POUND mnemonic:
    - Pulsatile
    - One-day duration (minimum 4 hours)
    - Unilateral
    - Nausea/vomiting
    - Disabling intensity

PRACTICE

The most predictive features for distinguishing migraine from tension-type headaches are nausea, photophobia, phonophobia, exacerbation by physical activity, and aura.

Evidence

- **Source:** Smetana GW. The diagnostic value of historical features in primary headache syndromes: a comprehensive review. *Arch Intern Med.* 2000;160(18):2729–37.
- **Takeaways:**
  - Nausea, photophobia, phonophobia, exacerbation by physical activity, and aura were the best differentiators from tension-type headache and had positive likelihood ratios of ranging from 3.7 to 19.2.
- **Notes:**
  - Cluster headaches are strictly unilateral.

PRACTICE

Severe migraines are acutely treated with triptans or triptan-NSAID combinations.

Evidence

- **Source:** Lipton RB, Bigal ME, Goadsby PJ. Double-blind clinical trials of oral triptans vs other classes of acute migraine medication—a review. *Cephalalgia.* 2004;24:321–332.
- **Takeaways:**
  - In a meta-analysis of nine double-blind RCTs comparing an oral triptan to a different abortive medication class in treatment of acute migraine, increased efficacy of triptans was underwhelming.
- **Source:** Brandes JL, Kudrow D, Stark SR, et al. Sumatriptan-naproxen for acute treatment of migraine: a randomized trial. *JAMA.* 2007;297(13):1443–54.
- **Takeaways:**
  - Sumatriptan-naproxen demonstrated 9% better efficacy at reducing pain secondary to migraine than lone sumatriptan therapy.
- **Notes:**
  - Although triptans have not been convincingly demonstrated to have greater efficacy than other classes of abortive medications for acute headache, clinical experience suggests otherwise and many of the studies have been underpowered. Hence most clinicians continue to use standalone triptan therapy as escalation step after NSAIDs.
  - Triptans primarily target 5HT1b and 5HT1d receptors (same receptors as ergotamines but more specific).

PRACTICE

Calcitonin gene–related peptide (CGRP) inhibitors may be used as prophylactic therapy for migraines.

Evidence

- **Source:** Silberstein SD, Dodick DW, Bigal ME, et al. Fremanezumab for the preventive treatment of chronic migraine. *N Engl J Med.* 2017;377:2113–22.
- **Takeaways:**
  - CGRP inhibitor use significantly decreased (4 to 4.5 days) headache frequency.
- **Notes:**
  - Due to the recent approval and cost, CGRP inhibitors are not first or second line therapy and are used for chronic refractory migraines.

PRACTICE

Migraine with aura is a contraindication to the use of estrogen-containing contraceptives.

Evidence

- **Source:** Chang CL, Donaghy M, Poulter N. Migraine and stroke in young women: case-control study. The World Health Organisation Collaborative Study of Cardiovascular Disease and Steroid Hormone Contraception. *BMJ.* 1999;318(7175):13–8.
- **Takeaways:**
  - In young women taking estrogen-containing oral contraceptives, the risk of ischemic but not hemorrhagic stroke is increased (odds ratio [OR] 3.54).
- **Notes:**
  - Progesterone-only contraceptives may be used as they have not been shown to increase the risk of stroke.

PRACTICE

NSAIDs are the mainstay of therapy for acute abortive treatment of tension headaches.

Evidence

- **Source:** Verhagen AP, Damen L, Berger MY, et al. Treatment of tension headache: paracetamol and NSAIDs work: a systematic review. *Ned Tijdschr Geneeskd.* 2010;154:A1924.
- **Takeaways:**
  - Meta-analysis showed increased efficacy (relative risk 1.3) of NSAIDs compared with acetaminophen.
  - No difference in efficacy of various NSAIDs
- **Notes:**
  - If NSAIDs or acetaminophen does not provide relief of tension headache, try maximizing the dose prior to switching medication class.

PRACTICE

Tricyclic antidepressants (TCAs), particularly amitriptyline, are first-line therapy as preventative medications for tension-type headaches.

Evidence

- **Source:** Jackson JL, Mancuso JM, Nickoloff S, et al. Tricyclic and tetracyclic antidepressants for the prevention of frequent episodic or chronic tension-type headache in adults: a systematic review and meta-analysis. *J Gen Intern Med.* 2017;32(12):1351–8.
- **Takeaways:**
  - TCAs were superior to placebo in reducing frequency of tension headaches.
  - TCAs were more effective than selective serotonin reuptake inhibitors.
- **Notes:**
  - Check carefully for cardiovascular conditions that may prohibit use of TCAs.

PRACTICE

First line therapy for acute abortion of cluster headache is oxygen.

Evidence

- **Source:** Petersen AS, Barloese MCJ, Jensen RH. Oxygen treatment of cluster headache: a review. *Cephalalgia.* 2014;34(13):1079–87.
- **Takeaways:**
  - Low-flow (6 to 7 L/min) oxygen therapy is effective in aborting cluster headaches.
- **Notes:**
  - Oxygen therapy is one of the few examples of an ideal treatment because it is highly effective without side effects.

Transient Ischemic Attack/Stroke

PRACTICE

The National Institute of Health Stroke Scale (NIHSS) is the leading 15-question survey for assessment of acute stroke severity.

Evidence

- **Source:** Brott T, Adams HP Jr, Olinger CP, et al. Measurements of acute cerebral infarction: a clinical examination scale. *Stroke.* 1989;20:864–70.
- **Takeaways:**
  - This is the original paper that published the NIHSS as a means of categorizing strokes by severity in stroke therapy trials.
  - High interrater reliability and test-retest reliability
- **Notes:**
  - Classification of severity is useful for determining specific interventions, such as decreasing the tissue plasminogen activator (tPA) window to 3 hours.

PRACTICE

The NIHSS is validated for quick classification of the severity and likelihood of an acute stroke.

Evidence

- **Source:** Adams HP Jr, Davis PH, Leira EC, et al. Baseline NIH Stroke Scale score strongly predicts outcome after stroke: a report of the Trial of Org 10172 in Acute Stroke Treatment (TOAST). *Neurology.* 1999;53(1):126.
- **Takeaways:**

- NIHSS of 16 or greater predicts high mortality and morbidity.
- NIHSS of 6 or less predicts good recovery.
- Each additional point on the NIHSS decreases the likelihood of excellent outcomes at 7 days by 24%.
- **Notes:**
  - It is very important to understand a patient's baseline prior to the current acute event. For example, does the patient have preexisting weakness or paralysis? Blindness? Dysarthria?

PRACTICE

The baseline NIHSS upon admission has a strong correlation with outcomes at 1 year.

Evidence

- **Source:** Appelros P, Terént A. Characteristics of the National Institute of Health Stroke Scale: results from a population-based stroke cohort at baseline and after one year. *Cerebrovasc Dis.* 2004;17:21–7.
- **Takeaways:**
  - At 1 year, 75% of patients with NIHSS less than 4 were functionally independent.
  - Predictors of poor outcome were increased age and decreased consciousness.
- **Notes:**
  - Understanding prognosis early can help with efforts to provide specific interventions.

PRACTICE

The modified NIHSS (mNIHSS) is a 10-question survey for assessment of neurologic impairment by acute stroke.

Evidence

- **Source:** Lyden PD, Lu M, Levine SR, et al.; NINDS rtPA Stroke Study Group. A modified National Institutes of Health Stroke Scale for use in stroke clinical trials: preliminary reliability and validity. *Stroke.* 2001;32:1310–7.
- **Takeaways:**
  - mNIHSS was noninferior to the NIHSS in terms of validity and interrater reliability.
- **Notes:**
  - The mNIHSS has been shown in subsequent studies to have superior interrater reliability.

PRACTICE

The TOAST stroke classification is the leading definition used for achieving consistency across ischemic stroke therapy trials.

Evidence

- **Source:** TOAST Trial. Adams HP Jr, Bendixen BH, Kappelle LJ, et al. Classification of subtype of acute ischemic stroke. Definitions for use in a multicenter clinical trial. TOAST. Trial of Org 10172 in Acute Stroke Treatment. *Stroke.* 1993;24:35–41.
- **Takeaways:**
  - Very high interphysician agreement of stroke type
- **Notes:**
  - There are five subtypes of stroke under the TOAST classification:
    - Large-artery atherosclerosis

- Cardioembolism
- Small-vessel occlusion
- Stroke of other determined etiology
- Stroke of undetermined etiology

PRACTICE

The CHADSVASc score is used in patients with nonvalvular atrial fibrillation to risk stratify for thromboembolic stroke and decide on necessity of anticoagulation.

Evidence

- **Source:** Lip GYH, Nieuwlaat R, Pisters R, et al. Refining clinical risk stratification for predicting stroke and thromboembolism in atrial fibrillation using a novel risk factor-based approach. *Chest.* 2010;137(2):263–72.
- **Takeaways:**
  - Original study suggesting improved predictive value of the CHADSVASc score for thromboembolic stroke compared with the CHADS2 score
- **Source:** Friberg L, Rosenqvist M, Lip GYH. Evaluation of risk stratification schemes for ischaemic stroke and bleeding in 182 678 patients with atrial fibrillation: the Swedish Atrial Fibrillation cohort study. *Eur Heart J.* 2012;33(12):1500–10.
- **Takeaways:**
  - Verification of the CHADSVASc score in the Swedish Atrial Fibrillation cohort study
- **Notes:**
  - The score pertains only to **nonvalvular** atrial fibrillation.
  - The emphasis on the sex variable has been less, with recommendations that antithrombotic therapy not be given if the score is 1 due to female gender.

PRACTICE

Forearm rolling is used as a quick exam maneuver that can elicit subtle motor weakness.

Evidence

- **Source:** Sawyer RN Jr, Hanna JP, Ruff RL, Leigh RJ. Asymmetry of forearm rolling as a sign of unilateral cerebral dysfunction. *Neurology.* 1993;43:1596–8.
- **Takeaways:**
  - 87.1% sensitivity and 100% specificity for unilateral cerebral lesion
  - Most sensitive exam maneuver among others such as pronator drift, finger tapping, Babinski
- **Notes:**
  - Finger rolling is a variant of the forearm roll that can elicit even subtler weakness.

PRACTICE

The most sensitive imaging modality for stroke is diffusion-weighted imaging (DWI).

Evidence

- **Source:** Sorensen AG, Buonanno FS, Gonzalez RG, et al. Hyperacute stroke: evaluation with combined multisection diffusion-weighted and hemodynamically weighted echoplanar MR imaging. *Radiology.* 1996;199:2:391–401.

- **Takeaways:**
  - Ischemic injury of the brain is depicted earlier on DWI than CT or MRI.
- **Notes:**
  - DWI is based upon the restricted diffusion of water molecules. Water shifts occur very soon after ischemic stroke, hence the very early detection of acute ischemic injury as early as 3 minutes after onset.

PRACTICE

Thrombolysis using tPA within 3 hours of onset of acute ischemic stroke lowers mortality and neurologic morbidity.

Evidence

- **Source:** The National Institute of Neurological Disorders and Stroke rt-PA Stroke Study Group. Tissue plasminogen activator for acute ischemic stroke. *N Engl J Med.* 1995;333:1581–8.
- **Takeaways:**
  - tPA use was 30% more likely to yield minimal or no neurologic disability at 3 months.
  - Increased symptomatic intracerebral hemorrhage with tPA administration (6.4% vs. 0.6%)
- **Notes:**
  - Always rule out contraindications to tPA administration! Common exclusion criteria include:
    - Active bleeding anywhere
    - Prior history of intracranial bleeding
    - Significant head trauma in prior 3 months
    - Transient ischemic attack (TIA)/stroke in prior 3 months
    - Systolic blood pressure (SBP) greater than 185 or diastolic blood pressure (DBP) greater than 110
    - Active anticoagulation (warfarin, direct oral anticoagulants)
    - Arteriovenous malformation (AVM)
    - Intracranial neoplasm

PRACTICE

Under stricter exclusion criteria, tPA may be administered up to 4.5 hours after onset of acute ischemic stroke.

Evidence

- **Source:** Lees KR, Bluhmki E, von Kummer R, et al. Time to treatment with intravenous alteplase and outcome in stroke: an updated pooled analysis of ECASS, ATLANTIS, NINDS, and EPITHET trials. *Lancet.* 2010;375(9727):1695–703.
- **Takeaways:**
  - Favorable 3-month outcomes with thrombolysis seen up to 4.5 hours after symptom onset
  - 5.2% risk of significant intracranial hemorrhage with alteplase administration
- **Source:** NINDS Trial. National Institute of Neurological Disorders and Stroke rt-PA Stroke Study Group. Tissue plasminogen activator for acute ischemic stroke. *N Engl J Med.* 1995;333:1581–8.

- **Takeaways:**
  - In acute ischemic stroke, thrombolysis up to 3 hours improved neurologic outcomes but not mortality.
- **Source:** ECASS III Trial. Hacke W, Kaste M, Bluhmki E, et al.; ECASS Investigators. Thrombolysis with alteplase 3 to 4.5 hours after acute ischemic stroke. *N Engl J Med.* 2008;359:1317–29.
- **Takeaways:**
  - First trial to demonstrate improved functional outcomes but not mortality at 3 months with thrombolysis beyond 3 hours (up to 4.5 hours)
  - Greatest benefit was seen for thrombolysis within 90 minutes of symptom onset.
- **Notes:**
  - Administration after 3 hours but before 4.5 hours of stroke onset has these additional contraindications:
    - NIHSS greater than 25
    - Age greater than 80
    - Stroke greater than 1/3 of middle cerebral artery territory

PRACTICE

Hypertension during acute ischemic TIA/stroke is not treated unless blood pressure is greater than 220/120.

Evidence

- **Source:** Semplicini A, Maresca A, Boscolo G, et al. Hypertension in acute ischemic stroke: a compensatory mechanism or an additional damaging factor? *Arch Intern Med.* 2003;163(2):211–6.
- **Takeaways:**
  - Stroke outcomes were best in patients with higher SBPs, with 220 mm Hg being the highest in this study cohort.
- **Notes:**
  - Labetalol is first line for lowering SBPs greater than 220 mm Hg.

PRACTICE

In an active hemorrhagic stroke, SBP is lowered quickly to less than 140 mm Hg.

Evidence

- **Source:** INTERACT Trial. Anderson CS, Huang Y, Wang JG, et al.; INTERACT Investigators. Intensive blood pressure reduction in acute cerebral haemorrhage trial (INTERACT): a randomised pilot trial. *Lancet.* 2008;7(6):391–9.
- **Takeaways:**
  - Hematoma growth was reduced with intensive blood pressure control.
  - No change in adverse events or secondary clinical outcomes
- **Notes:**
  - Any coagulopathies should be corrected immediately in hemorrhagic stroke.

PRACTICE

Aspirin 325 mg is initiated within 24 to 48 hours of ischemic stroke.

Evidence

- **Source:** IST Trial. IST Collaborative Group. The International Stroke Trial (IST): a randomised trial of aspirin, subcutaneous heparin, both, or neither among 19435 patients with acute ischaemic stroke. *Lancet.* 1997;349(9065):1569–81.
- **Takeaways:**
  - Trend towards reduced mortality and neurologic disability at 6 months
  - Significantly fewer recurrent ischemic strokes (28%) or death (9%) in 14 days with no increase in hemorrhagic strokes
- **Notes:**
  - A larger trial known as the Chinese Acute Stroke Trial demonstrated similar findings.

PRACTICE

Standard secondary stroke prevention includes daily baby aspirin (81 mg).

Evidence

- **Source:** Antithrombotic Trialists' Collaboration. Collaborative meta-analysis of randomised trials of antiplatelet therapy for prevention of death, myocardial infarction, and stroke in high risk patients. *BMJ.* 2002;324:71.
- **Takeaways:**
  - Aspirin use significantly decreased vascular events (25%), nonfatal myocardial infarction (33%), nonfatal stroke (25%), and vascular mortality.
  - Higher doses of aspirin were equally as effective as low doses (75 to 150 mg).
- **Notes:**
  - Always consider potential bleeding risks prior to aspirin use.

PRACTICE

Dual antiplatelet therapy (DAPT) with aspirin and clopidogrel is used for secondary stroke prevention in acute minor stroke or TIA.

Evidence

- **Source:** ACTIVE A Trial. ACTIVE Investigators; Connolly SJ, Pogue J, Hart RG, et al. Effect of clopidogrel added to aspirin in patients with atrial fibrillation. *N Engl J Med.* 2009;360(20):2066–78.
- **Takeaways:**
  - DAPT reduced the rate (0.9% absolute reduction) of vascular events, particularly stroke, compared with aspirin alone.
  - Increased rate of major hemorrhage
- **Source:** CHANCE Trial. Wang Y, Wang Y, Zhao X, et al.; CHANCE Investigators. Clopidogrel with aspirin in acute minor stroke or transient ischemic attack. *N Engl J Med.* 2013;369:11–9.
- **Takeaways:**
  - DAPT with Clopidogrel was superior (3.5%) to monotherapy with aspirin in preventing stroke within 90 days of initial onset when NIHSS less than 4 or TIA.
  - No increase in rates of bleeding or hemorrhagic stroke conversion
- **Notes:**
  - No benefit found in other studies for DAPT for moderate-severe strokes.

PRACTICE

Patients with atrial fibrillation and CHADSVASc scores of 2 or greater are anticoagulated for risk reduction of stroke.

Evidence

- **Source:** SPAF Trial. SPAF Investigators. Stroke Prevention in Atrial Fibrillation Study. *Circulation.* 1991;84:527–39.
- **Takeaways:**
  - In nonvalvular atrial fibrillation, both warfarin and aspirin had a relative risk reduction (67% and 42%, respectively) in stroke.
  - No direct comparison of warfarin versus aspirin
- **Source:** ACTIVE W Trial. ACTIVE Writing Group of the ACTIVE Investigators; Connolly S, Pogue J, Hart R, et al. Clopidogrel plus aspirin versus oral anticoagulation for atrial fibrillation in the Atrial fibrillation Clopidogrel Trial with Irbesartan for prevention of Vascular Events (ACTIVE W): a randomised controlled trial. *Lancet.* 2006;367(9526):1903–12.
- **Takeaways:**
  - In nonvalvular atrial fibrillation, anticoagulation with warfarin was superior to antiplatelet therapy in preventing vascular events, including stroke.
  - Similar bleeding rates between DAPT and warfarin
- **Notes:**
  - SPAF was the first study to open the doors to anticoagulation for prevention of stroke.

PRACTICE

High-intensity statins are first line therapy for secondary stroke prevention.

Evidence

- **Source:** SPARCL Trial. High-dose atorvastatin after stroke or transient ischemic attack. *N Engl J Med.* 2006;355:549–59.
- **Takeaways:**
  - 1.9% reduction in fatal or nonfatal stroke
  - 3.5% absolute reduction in cardiovascular events
  - Slight increase in hemorrhagic stroke
  - No difference in mortality
- **Notes:**
  - High-intensity statins should be used carefully in the elderly or substituted with moderate-intensity statins.
  - Care should be taken when combining statins with fibrates (although combined use with fenofibrate has a lower risk of statin myopathy).
  - High-intensity statin regimens
    - Atorvastatin 40 to 80 mg
    - Rosuvastatin 20 to 40 mg
  - Moderate-intensity statin regimens
    - Atorvastatin 10 to 20 mg
    - Rosuvastatin 5 to 10 mg
    - Simvastatin 20 to 40 mg
    - Lovastatin 40 mg
    - Pravastatin 40 to 80 mg

PRACTICE

Fluoxetine is occasionally used for motor recovery in ischemic stroke with hemiparesis/plegia.

Evidence

- **Source:** FLAME Trial. Chollet F, Tardy J, Albucher JF, et al. Fluoxetine for motor recovery after acute ischaemic stroke (FLAME): a randomised placebo-controlled trial. *Lancet Neurol.* 2011;10(2):123–30.
- **Takeaways:**
  - Improved motor recovery in moderate-severe ischemic stroke after 3 months
- **Notes:**
  - Main adverse effects of fluoxetine include hyponatremia and gastrointestinal (GI) symptoms.

PRACTICE

Carotid endarterectomy (CEA) is recommended for significant carotid stenosis in the setting of TIA/stroke.

Evidence

- **Source:** NASCET Trial. Barnett HJ, Taylor DW, Eliasziw M, et al. Benefit of carotid endarterectomy in patients with symptomatic moderate or severe stenosis. North American Symptomatic Carotid Endarterectomy Trial Collaborators. *N Engl J Med.* 1998;339(20):1415–1425.
- **Takeaways:**
  - CEA reduced the 5-year risk of death or stroke by 29% for carotid stenosis greater than 50%.
  - Severe stenosis of 70% or greater had a significant reduction in stroke at 8-year follow-up.
  - No significant benefit for stenosis less than 50%
- **Source:** ECST Trial. ECST Group. Randomised trial of endarterectomy for recently symptomatic carotid stenosis: final results of the MRC European Carotid Surgery Trial (ECST). *Lancet.* 1998;351(9113):1379–87.
- **Takeaways:**
  - CEA significantly reduced mortality and recurrent stroke rates (14.9% vs. 26.5%) in carotid stenosis of 80% or greater.
- **Source:** North American Symptomatic Carotid Endarterectomy Trial Collaborators; Barnett HJM, Taylor DW, Haynes RB, et al. Beneficial effect of carotid endarterectomy in symptomatic patients with high-grade carotid stenosis. *N Engl J Med.* 1991;325:445–53.
- **Takeaways:**
  - Among severe stenosis (≥70%), 17% absolute risk reduction in ipsilateral stroke
- **Notes:**
  - Many experts believe that the benefits and risks of CEA highly depend on surgical skill.
  - Difference between stenosis degree required to benefit between NASCET and ECST trials may be related to different methods of measuring the stenoses.

PRACTICE

CEA is preferred versus stenting in patients with 60% or greater stenosis, whereas CEA and stenting are based on patient profile (age, difficult carotid anatomy) for stenosis of 70% or greater.

Evidence

- **Source:** EVA-3S Trial. Mas JL, Chatellier G, Beyssen B, et al.; EVA-3S Investigators. Endarterectomy versus stenting in patients with symptomatic severe carotid stenosis. *N Engl J Med.* 2006;355:1660–71.
- **Takeaways:**
  - Significantly greater risk of stroke or mortality (relative risk 2.5) with stenting versus endarterectomy for stenosis of 60% or greater.
- **Source:** CREST Trial. Brott TG, Hobson RW 2nd, Howard G, et al.; CREST Investigators. Stenting versus endarterectomy for treatment of carotid-artery stenosis. *N Engl J Med.* 2010;363(1):11–23.
- **Takeaways:**
  - No difference between CEA and stenting for stroke, myocardial infarction, or mortality at 4 years
  - Stenting associated with lower periprocedural rates of myocardial infarction
  - CEA associated with lower periprocedural rates of stroke
- **Notes:**
  - CEA carries a higher risk of cranial nerve damage and systemic (pulmonary) complications, but differences have not been found to be statistically significant.

PRACTICE

Patent foramen ovale (PFO) closure is superior to medical therapy for prevention of recurrent cryptogenic stroke.

Evidence

- **Source:** REDUCE Trial. Søndergaard L, Kasner SE, Rhodes JF, et al.; Gore REDUCE Clinical Study Investigators. Patent foramen ovale closure or antiplatelet therapy for cryptogenic stroke. *N Engl J Med.* 2017;377:1033–1042.
- **Source:** CLOSE Trial. Mas JL, Derumeaux G, Guillon B, et al.; CLOSE Investigators. Patent foramen ovale closure or anticoagulation vs. antiplatelets after stroke. *N Engl J Med.* 2017;377:1011–1021.
- **Takeaways:**
  - PFO closure significantly decreased recurrent stroke risk compared with antiplatelet therapy (ranging from 3.5% to 4% absolute reduction).
  - Increased risk of atrial fibrillation and venous thromboembolism
- **Notes:**
  - In prior trials, PFO closure has not shown a statistically significant benefit, but the studies had many flaws, including the inclusion of patients who would not benefit from PFO closure.

PRACTICE

Thrombectomy is recommended for patients who present with ischemic stroke secondary to a large vessel occlusion up to 24 hours.

Evidence

- **Source:** DAWN Trial. Nogueira RG, Jadhav AP, Haussen DC, et al.; DAWN Trial Investigators. Thrombectomy 6 to 24 hours after stroke with a mismatch between deficit and infarct. *N Engl J Med.* 2018;378(1):11–21.

- **Takeaways:**
  - Thrombectomy significantly improved functional outcomes at 90 days.
  - No difference in symptomatic intracranial hemorrhage
- **Notes:**
  - There are several eligibility criteria that should be checked prior to thrombectomy in qualifying patients.

Head Trauma

PRACTICE

The Canadian Head CT rules are a common tool for identifying patients for head CT necessary in the setting of acute head trauma.

Evidence

- **Source:** Stielli IG, Wells GA, Vandemheen K, et al. The Canadian CT head rule for patients with minor head injury. *Lancet.* 2001;357(9266):1391–6.
- **Source:** Stielli IG, Clement CM, Rowe BH, et al. Comparison of the Canadian CT head rule and the New Orleans criteria in patients with minor head injury. *JAMA.* 2005;294(12):1511–8.
- **Takeaways:**
  - Rules are stratified into high-risk (to rule out need for neurosurgical intervention) and moderate-risk (to rule out clinically significant brain injury) criteria.
  - 100% sensitivity for need for neurosurgical intervention and clinically important brain injuries
- **Notes:**
  - The Canadian Head CT rules have been shown in several studies to reduce the rate of head CT imaging by approximately 30%.
  - The New Orleans Criteria have been shown consistently to have lower sensitivity than the CHCT rules.
  - Exclusion criteria:
    - Age less than 16
    - Patient on anticoagulation
    - Seizure after injury

Seizures

PRACTICE

Standard work-up for an unprovoked first-time seizure includes electroencephalogram and MRI (CT if MRI unavailable).

Evidence

- **Source:** Harden CL, Huff JS, Schwartz TH, et al. Reassessment: neuroimaging in the emergency patient presenting with seizure (an evidence-based review): report of the Therapeutics and Technology Assessment Subcommittee of the American Academy of Neurology. *Neurology.* 2007;69:1772–80.
- **Takeaways:**
  - Management for adults with unprovoked first-time seizures changed in 9% to 17% of cases.

- **Notes:**
  - Risk factors such as human immunodeficiency virus (HIV)/acquired immunodeficiency syndrome (AIDS) increase the likelihood of clinically significant abnormal imaging findings.

PRACTICE

Lorazepam is the first-line therapy for status epilepticus.

Evidence

- **Source:** Alldredge BK, Gelb AM, Isaacs SM, et al. A comparison of lorazepam, diazepam, and placebo for the treatment of out-of-hospital status epilepticus. *N Engl J Med.* 2001;345:631–7.
- **Takeaways:**
  - Lorazepam had the highest termination of status epilepticus (59.1%) versus diazepam (42.6%).
- **Notes:**
  - Lorazepam is also useful in patients with liver dysfunction, because it is mostly metabolized by conjugation.

PRACTICE

Levetiracetam and phenytoin are both second line agents for status epilepticus.

Evidence

- **Source:** EcLiPSE Trial. Lyttle MD, Rainford NEA, Gamble C, et al.; Paediatric Emergency Research in the United Kingdom & Ireland (PERUKI) collaborative. Levetiracetam versus phenytoin for second-line treatment of paediatric convulsive status epilepticus (EcLiPSE): a multicentre, open-label, randomised trial. *Lancet.* 2019;393(10186):2125–34.
- **Takeaways:**
  - No significant difference between levetiracetam and phenytoin for termination of status epilepticus
- **Notes:**
  - Levetiracetam is often favored due to a better side effect profile and faster infusion time.
  - Data suggest that fosphenytoin, levetiracetam, and valproate are equally effective.

PRACTICE

In the absence of abnormal head imaging or EEG, first-time seizures do not warrant antiepileptic therapy.

Evidence

- **Source:** Marson A, Jacoby A, Johnson A, et al. Immediate versus deferred antiepileptic drug treatment for early epilepsy and single seizures: a randomised controlled trial. *Lancet.* 2005;365(9476):2007–13.
- **Takeaways:**
  - No difference in seizure prevalence at 5-year follow-up
  - Antiepileptic treatment increased the time to first seizure.
- **Notes:**
  - The antiepileptic with the least side effects is levetiracetam (Keppra).

PRACTICE

Levetiracetam is first line therapy for partial seizures.

Evidence

- **Source:** Cereghino JJ, Biton V, Abou-Khalil B, et al. Levetiracetam for partial seizures: results of a double-blind, randomized clinical trial. *Neurology.* 2000;55(2):236–42.
- **Source:** Shorvon SD, Löwenthal A, Janz D, et al. Multicenter double-blind, randomized, placebo-controlled trial of levetiracetam as add-on therapy in patients with refractory partial seizures. European Levetiracetam Study Group. *Epilepsia.* 2000;41(9):1179–86.
- **Source:** Ben-Menachem E, Falter U. Efficacy and tolerability of levetiracetam 3000 mg/day in patients with refractory partial seizures: a multicenter, double-blind, responder-selected study evaluating monotherapy. European Levetiracetam Study Group. *Epilepsia.* 2000;41(10):1276–83.
- **Takeaways:**
  - Three trials demonstrated the high efficacy and good tolerability of levetiracetam for partial seizures.
- **Notes:**
  - Compared with other antiepileptics, levetiracetam can be used for a wider range of seizure types and has fewer side effects.
  - Most common side effects of levetiracetam:
    - Headache
    - Asthenia
    - Somnolence
    - Mood effects

Meningitis

Practice

Dexamethasone should be initiated as soon as possible along with antibiotics for suspected bacterial meningitis.

Evidence

- **Source:** de Gans JD, van de Beek D; European Dexamethasone in Adulthood Bacterial Meningitis Study Investigators. Dexamethasone in adults with bacterial meningitis. *N Engl J Med.* 2002;347(20):1549–56.
- **Takeaways:**
  - 52% mortality benefit and 41% Glasgow Outcome Scale benefit with adjunctive dexamethasone therapy in bacterial meningitis
  - Benefits were largely driven by *Streptococcus pneumonia.*
- **Notes:**
  - Dexamethasone therapy is primarily intended for *S. pneumonia* meningitis, but due to the necessity to administer early prior to diagnostic confirmation of the organism, it is practically administered for most bacterial meningitis cases.

PRACTICE

Head CT should be obtained prior to lumbar puncture in meningitis patients with certain risk factors to screen for increased mass effect and prevent rare but fatal herniation.

Evidence

- **Source:** Hasbun R, et al. Computed tomography of the head before lumbar puncture in adults with suspected meningitis. *N Engl J Med.* 2001;345(24):1727–33.
- **Takeaways:**
  - Various features were found to increase likelihood of abnormal head CT imaging in meningitis patients:
    - Age greater than 60
    - Immunocompromise
    - Seizure prior to presentation
    - History of central nervous system disease
    - Altered mental status
- **Notes:**
  - An early sign of herniation is ocular palsies, particularly abducens or oculomotor palsy.

PRACTICE

Meningitis is typically thought of as the triad of fever, altered mental status, and stiff neck. However, it is more common to not have the triad in acute bacterial meningitis.

Evidence

- **Source:** Van de Beek D, de Gans J, Spanjaard L, et al. Clinical features and prognostic factors in adults with bacterial meningitis. *N Engl J Med.* 2004;351(18):1849.
- **Takeaways:**
  - The classic meningitis triad was found only in 44% of acute bacterial meningitis cases.
  - Most patients (95%) had at least two of four symptoms: fever, headache, neck stiffness, altered mental status.
- **Notes:**
  - The classic meningitis triad is more commonly found in elderly patients.

Neuromuscular Disorders

PRACTICE

Acetylcholinesterase inhibiters are routinely used for treatment of myasthenia gravis.

Evidence

- **Source:** Mehndiratta MM, Pandey S, Kuntzer T. Acetylcholinesterase inhibitor treatment for myasthenia gravis. *Cochrane Database Syst Rev.* 2014;2014(10):CD006986.
- **Takeaways:**
  - Observational studies provide very strong evidence for the effectiveness of acetylcholinesterase inhibitors in the treatment of myasthenia gravis.
  - No significant RCTs that have explored the effectiveness of acetylcholinesterase inhibitors for myasthenia gravis
- **Notes:**
  - Myasthenia gravis impacts the nicotinic postsynaptic receptors at the neuromuscular junction.

PRACTICE

The ice-pack test is a quick test for detecting subtle myasthenia gravis.

Evidence

- **Source:** Golnik KC, Pena R, Lee AG, Eggenberger ER. An ice test for the diagnosis of myasthenia gravis. *Ophthalmology.* 1999;106(7):1282.
- **Takeaways:**
  - 80% sensitivity for myasthenia gravis in patients with incomplete ptosis
- **Notes:**
  - The edrophonium test is no longer used in the United States due to risk of potentiating muscarinic effects, which are particularly dangerous in patients with cardiovascular disease.
  - This test may be uncomfortable for the patient (imagine having ice on your eyes for 2 minutes)!

PRACTICE

Anti-MuSK (muscle-specific kinase) is a serologic test for detecting myasthenia gravis.

Evidence

- **Source:** Lavrnic D, Losen M, Vujic A, et al. The features of myasthenia gravis with auto-antibodies to MuSK. *J Neurol Neurosrug Psychiatry.* 2005;76(8):1099.
- **Takeaways:**
  - Present in 38% to 50% of myasthenia gravis patients negative for AChR-Ab (anti-acetylcholinesterase receptor antibody)
  - Anti-MuSK was found almost exclusively in female patients.
  - Patients with anti-MuSK usually (82.4%) had facial and bulbar muscle involvement.
- **Notes:**
  - More studies are beginning to elicit differences in features and prognosis based on the presence of varying antibodies, including anti-MuSK.

PRACTICE

First line therapies for Guillain-Barré syndrome include plasmapheresis and intravenous immunoglobulin therapy.

Evidence

- **Source:** Patwa HS, Chaudhry V, Katzberg H, et al. Evidence-based guideline: intravenous immunoglobulin in the treatment of neuromuscular disorders: report of the Therapeutics and Technology Assessment Subcommittee of the American Academy of Neurology. *Neurology.* 2012;78(13):1009.
- **Takeaways:**
  - Either plasmapheresis or IVIG is effective in treating acute Guillain-Barré syndrome.
  - No benefit to combining both IVIG and plasmapheresis
- **Notes:**
  - Plasmapheresis requires dialysis access and thus is more difficult to undertake.

Movement Disorders
PRACTICE

In early Parkinson disease, monoamine oxidase type B (MAO-B) inhibitors may be an effective therapy.

Evidence

- **Source:** Ives NJ, Stowe RL, Marro J, et al. Monoamine oxidase type B inhibitors in early Parkinson's disease: meta-analysis of 17 randomised trials involving 3525 patients. *BMJ.* 2004;329(7466):593.
- **Takeaways:**
  - MAO-B inhibitors demonstrated small improvements in motor scores, motor fluctuations, and need for levodopa in 1 year.
- **Notes:**
  - MAO-B inhibitors should be avoided with diets high in tyramine (cheese, aged wine) due to risk of hypertensive crisis.

PRACTICE

In early tremor-predominant Parkinson disease, amantadine may be a good alternative to MAO B inhibitors.

Evidence

- **Source:** Schwab RS, Poskanzer DC, England AC Jr, Young RR. Amantadine in Parkinson's disease: review of more than two years' experience. *JAMA.* 1972;222(7):792–5.
- **Takeaways:**
  - Significant improvement in two-thirds of patients on amantadine and four-fifths of patients on amantadine with levodopa
- **Notes:**
  - Subsequent trials have shown that amantadine is superior to anticholinergics for bradykinesia and rigidity.

PRACTICE

Anticholinergics are used as ancillary treatment in Parkinson disease, particularly for improving motor function.

Evidence

- **Source:** Katzenschlager R, Sampaio C, Costa J, Lees A. Anticholinergics for symptomatic management of Parkinson's disease. *Cochrane Database Syst Rev.* 2003;(2):CD003735.
- **Takeaways:**
  - Anticholinergics were superior to placebo in improving various aspects of Parkinson disease but particularly motor symptoms.
- **Notes:**
  - Be cautious of anticholinergics in patients older than 65 years, due to their side effects (most notably their neuropsychiatric and cognitive effects).

PRACTICE

Anticholinergics are ancillary treatments in Parkinson disease due to relatively lower efficacy than L-dopa.

Evidence

- **Source:** Parkes JD, Baxter RC, Marsden CD, Rees JE. Comparative trial of benzhexol, amantadine, and levodopa in the treatment of Parkinson's disease. *J Neurol Neurosurg Psychiatry.* 1974;37(4):422.

- **Takeaways:**
  - L-dopa had a 36% reduction in functional disability, whereas anticholinergics had a 15% reduction.
- **Notes:**
  - Despite the lower overall efficacy, anticholinergics are useful particularly in motor-predominant Parkinson disease.

PRACTICE

In early Parkinson disease, dopamine agonists are a viable therapeutic option.

Evidence

- **Source:** Stowe RL, Ives NJ, Clarke C, et al. Dopamine agonist therapy in early Parkinson's disease. *Cochrane Database Syst Rev.* 2008;(2):CD006564.
- **Takeaways:**
  - Dopamine agonists decreased dyskinesia, dystonia, and motor fluctuations (OR 0.43, 0.64, and 0.75, respectively).
- **Notes:**
  - Dopamine agonists may lead to nausea, orthostatic hypotension, and hallucinations as some of their most common side effects.

PRACTICE

L-dopa is the best long-term therapy for Parkinson disease.

Evidence

- **Source:** ELLDOPA Trial. Fahn S, Oakes D, Shoulson I, et al., Parkinson Study Group. Levodopa and the progression of Parkinson's disease. *N Engl J Med.* 2004;351:2498–508.
- **Takeaways:**
  - L-dopa was superior to placebo in reducing disease symptoms (>50% improvement compared with placebo on UPDRS scale).
    - This is not a trial comparing L-dopa to all other drug classes. Through natural history experiments and observation, rather than an RCT with direct comparisons, it has become without doubt that L-dopa is the best long-term therapy for Parkinson disease.
- **Notes:**
  - Avoid stopping L-dopa abruptly due to risk for malignant hyperthermia.
  - L-dopa is associated with higher risk for dyskinesia than other Parkinson drug classes.

PRACTICE

It is unclear whether Parkinson disease should be treated with alternatives to L-dopa first to maximize the duration of future L-dopa treatment (i.e., minimize development of resistance to L-dopa).

Evidence

- **Source:** ELLDOPA Trial. Fahn S, Oakes D, Shoulson I, et al.; Parkinson Study Group. Levodopa and the progression of Parkinson's disease. *N Engl J Med.* 2004;351:2498–508.
- **Takeaways:**
  - No clinical or imaging evidence for early L-dopa use and negative effects on long-term disease treatment/prognosis

- **Source:** Katzenschlager R, Head J, Schrag A, et al. Fourteen-year final report of the randomized PDRG-UK trial comparing three initial treatments in PD. *Neurology.* 2008;71(7):474–80.
- **Source:** Cilia R, Akpalu A, Sarfo FS, et al. The modern pre-levodopa era of Parkinson's disease: insights into motor complications from sub-Saharan Africa. *Brain.* 2014;137(Pt 10):2731–42.
- **Takeaways:**
  - Disease duration at time of L-dopa initiation was not associated with worse increased side effects.
- **Notes:**
  - Early thinking reflected a view of sparing L-dopa until it was truly needed (i.e., refractory disease to other therapies), but new evidence is demonstrating that the duration of therapy is less important than a patient's own unique physiology.

PRACTICE

Catechol-O-methyl-transferase (COMT) is not used in combination with L-dopa for early Parkinson therapy.

Evidence

- **Source:** Stocchi F, Rascol O, Kieburtz K, , et al. Initiating levodopa/carbidopa therapy with and without entacapone in early Parkinson disease: the STRIDE-PD study. *Ann Neurol.* 2010;68(1):18–27.
- **Takeaways:**
  - COMT inhibitor use led to earlier and more frequent dyskinesias than L-dopa monotherapy, without differences in motor improvement.
- **Notes:**
  - COMT inhibitors prevent degradation of L-dopa peripherally.

PRACTICE

Deep brain stimulation (DBS) may be effective for medication-refractory Parkinson disease, particularly the motor-predominant type.

Evidence

- **Source:** Deuschi G, Schade-Brittinger C, Krack P, et al., German Parkinson Study Group, Neurostimulation Section. A randomized trial of deep-brain stimulation for Parkinson's disease. *N Engl J Med.* 2006;355(9):896.
- **Takeaways:**
  - Quality of life was approximately 25% greater with DBS as opposed to maximal medical therapy.
  - 48% improvement in severity of symptoms without medications
- **Source:** Weaver FM, Follett K, Stern M, et al.; CSP 468 Study Group. Bilateral deep brain stimulation vs best medical therapy for patients with advanced Parkinson disease: a randomized controlled trial. *JAMA.* 2009;301(1):63.
- **Takeaways:**
  - Significant improvement in motor complications with DBS versus optimal medical therapy (dyskinesia free for 4.6 h/day more)
- **Notes:**
  - DBS placement heralds certain risks such as cognitive dysfunction and cerebral hemorrhage because the electrode passes through the cortex on its way to the basal ganglia.

PRACTICE

Propranolol and primidone are first line therapies for essential tremor.

Evidence

- **Source:** Gorman WP, Cooper R, Pocock P, Campbell MJ. A comparison of primidone, propranolol, and placebo in essential tremor, using quantitative analysis. *J Neurol Neurosurg Psychiatry.* 1986;49(1):64.
- **Takeaways:**
  - Both propranolol and primodine improved essential tremor by approximately 50%.
  - Patients with higher-frequency tremors responded to both drugs, whereas lower-frequency tremors responded to one or another.
- **Notes:**
  - Due to the side effect profile of primidone, many experts prefer propranolol.

PRACTICE

Primidone may be used to augment propranolol therapy in difficult-to-treat essential tremor.

Evidence

- **Source:** Koller WC, Royse VL. Efficacy of primidone in essential tremor. *Neurology.* 1986;36(1):121–4.
- **Takeaways:**
  - Addition of primidone to pronanolol led to a nearly 50% increase in reduction of tremor amplitude.
- **Notes:**
  - Primidone was originally developed as an anticonvulsant.

PRACTICE

Topiramate may be used for limb tremor in patients refractory to propranolol and primidone.

Evidence

- **Source:** Ondo WG, Jankovic J, Connor GS, et al.; Topiramate Essential Tremor Study Investigators. Topiramate in essential tremor: a double-blind, placebo-controlled trial. *Neurology.* 2006;66(5):672.
- **Takeaways:**
  - Topiramate improved tremor by 29% compared with placebo.
- **Notes:**
  - Most common side effects that limit topiramate therapy are paresthesias, nausea/vomiting, and decrease in concentration.

PRACTICE

DBS is sometimes used as treatment for refractory essential tremor.

Evidence

- **Source:** Zesiewicz TA, Elble R, Louis ED, et al.; Quality Standards Subcommittee of the American Academy of Neurology. Practice parameter: therapies for essential tremor: report of the Quality Standards Subcommittee of the American Academy of Neurology. *Neurology.* 2005;64(12):2008.

- **Takeaways:**
  - Review of the clinical trial literature regarding essential tremors from 1966 to 2004 suggested DBS is highly effective for reducing tremor despite a small risk of significant complications.
- **Notes:**
  - DBS lacks evidence for head and voice essential tremor treatment.

PRACTICE

Tetrabenazine is used to treat chorea in Huntington disease.

Evidence

- **Source:** Huntington Study Group. Tetrabenazine as antichorea therapy in Huntington disease: a randomized controlled trial. *Neurology.* 2006;66(3):366–72.
- **Takeaways:**
  - Tetrabenazine reduced chorea significantly more than placebo (unified Huntington's disease rating scale score difference of –5 vs. –1.5).
- **Notes:**
  - Tetrabenazine blocks the transport of dopamine into vesicles released in the presynaptic terminal, thereby decreasing excess dopamine-driven movement.

PRACTICE

Dopamine agonists are first-line therapy for restless leg syndrome (RLS).

Evidence

- **Takeaways:**
  - Dopamine agonists (particularly pramipexole and cabergoline) were superior in reducing RLS symptom severity compared with placebo.
- **Notes:**
  - RLS should be differentiated from peripheral neuropathy, which can present similarly.

PRACTICE

Gabapentin is a second line therapy for RLS.

Evidence

- **Source:** Lee DO, Ziman RB, Perkins AT, et al.; XP053 Study Group. A randomized, double-blind, placebo-controlled study to assess the efficacy and tolerability of gabapentin enacarbil in subjects with restless legs syndrome. *J Clin Sleep Med.* 2011;7(3):282–92.
- **Takeaways:**
  - Gabapentin was 32.7% more likely to alleviate RLS than was placebo.
- **Notes:**
  - Gabapentin is particularly useful for patients with RLS who also suffer from neuropathies.
  - First line therapy when patients have concomitant impulse control disorders

PRACTICE

Patients with RLS and anemia should have their iron repleted.

Evidence

- **Source:** Allen RP, Picchietti DL, Auerbach M, et al., International Restless Legs Syndrome Study Group (IRLSSG). Evidence-based and consensus clinical practice guidelines for the iron treatment of restless legs syndrome/Willis-Ekbom disease in adults and children: an IRLSSG task force report. *Sleep Med.* 2018;41:27.
- **Takeaways:**
  - Iron (intravenous > oral) may be effective in treating moderate to severe RLS in adults with ferritin of 75 µg/L or less.
- **Notes:**
  - Pica, a predilection for chewing ice, is a common sign of iron deficiency anemia.
  - Iron absorption increases when combined with vitamin C or orange juice (the ascorbic acid oxidizes iron to Fe^{3+}, which is the only form of iron absorbed).

Dementia

PRACTICE

The Montreal Cognitive Assessment (MOCA) is a commonly used screening tool for dementia

Evidence

- **Source:** Nasreddine ZS, Phillips NA, Bédirian V, et al. The Montreal Cognitive Assessment, MoCA: a brief screening tool for mild cognitive impairment. *J Am Geriatr Soc.* 2005;53(4):695.
- **Takeaways:**
  - Scores less than 26 detected 90% of mild cognitive impairment subjects.
  - 100% specific for detecting mild Alzheimer disease, as opposed to 87%
- **Notes:**
  - Many studies have demonstrated that the MOCA test is more difficult than the Mini-Mental Status Exam (MMSE).
  - Subsequent studies have suggested adding +1 to the overall score earned for formal education less than 12 years.

PRACTICE

The MMSE is a commonly used screening tool for dementia.

Evidence

- **Source:** Folstein MF, Folstein SE, McHugh PR. "Mini-mental state". A practical method for grading the cognitive state of patients for the clinician. *J Psychiatr Res.* 1975;12(3):189.
- **Takeaways:**
  - Scores less than 20 were associated only with dementia.
- **Source:** Tsoi KK, Chan JYC, Hirai HW, et al. Cognitive tests to detect dementia: a systematic review and meta-analysis. *JAMA Intern Med.* 2015;175(9):1450.
- **Takeaways:**
  - Pooled sensitivity and specificity of 81% and 89%, respectively
- **Notes:**
  - 30-point scale with varying cutoffs, generally with scores less than 24 considered cognitively impaired
  - Originally developed for assessment of psychiatric patients

PRACTICE

The Mini-Cog is a quick test used, often in primary care offices, to detect dementia.

Evidence

- **Source:** Borson S, Scanlan J, Brush M, et al. The mini-cog: a cognitive "vital signs" measure for dementia screening in multi-lingual elderly. *Int J Geriatr Psychiatry.* 2000;15(11):1021.
- **Takeaways:**
  - 99% sensitivity for dementia
- **Notes:**
  - Diagnostic value unaffected by education and language

PRACTICE

Acetylcholinesterase inhibitors are used for slowing the progress of Alzheimer disease.

Evidence

- **Source:** Birks J. Cholinesterase inhibitors for Alzheimer's disease. *Cochrane Database Syst Rev.* 2006;(1):CD005593.
- **Takeaways:**
  - Modest improvement of –2.7 points on the ADAS-Cog Scale with acetylcholinesterase inhibitors over 6- and 12-month periods
- **Notes:**
  - Severe dementia is classified as MMSE less than 10.

PRACTICE

N-methyl-D-aspartic acid inhibitors (in particular, memantine) are adjunctive therapies for **moderate to severe** Alzheimer disease.

Evidence

- **Source:** Reisberg B, Doody R, Stöffler A, et al.; Memantine Study Group. Memantine in moderate-to-severe Alzheimer's disease. *N Engl J Med* 2003;348(14):1333.
- **Takeaways:**
  - Significantly less clinical deterioration on multiple rating scales (CIBIC-Plus, Severe Impairment Battery, ADCS-ADLsev)
- **Source:** Howard R, McShane R, Lindesay J, et al. Donepezil and memantine for moderate-to-severe Alzheimer's disease. *N Engl J Med.* 2012;366(10):893–903.
- **Takeaways:**
  - Memantine addition to donepezil was superior to donepezil monotherapy in reducing cognitive impairment at a year in moderate-severe Alzheimer disease.
- **Notes:**
  - Do not use memantine for early disease!

PRACTICE

Vitamin E (2000 IU/day) is prescribed as a simple antioxidant therapy that may improve cognitive function and slow decline in Alzheimer disease.

Evidence

- **Source:** Sano M, Ernesto C, Thomas RG, et al. A controlled trial of selegiline, alpha-tocopherol, or both as treatment for Alzheimer's disease. The Alzheimer's Disease Cooperative Study. *N Engl J Med.* 1997;336(17):1216.
- **Takeaways:**
  - MMSE decline delayed by approximately 200 days with daily 2000 U vitamin E
  - Similar decline with vitamin E as with selegiline
- **Source:** Dysken MW, Sano M, Asthana S, et al. Effect of vitamin E and memantine on functional decline in Alzheimer disease: the TEAM-AD VA cooperative randomized trial. *JAMA.* 2014;311(1):33.
- **Takeaways:**
  - Vitamin E (2000 U/day) led to slower cognitive decline (ADCS-ADL) in patients with mild to moderate Alzheimer disease.
- **Notes:**
  - Signs of vitamin E toxicity include:
    - May block absorption of vitamin A or K
    - Decrease in vitamin K–dependent clotting factors (predisposed bleeding)
    - Vision changes
    - Some evidence to suggest increased mortality in patients with poor health who chronically live at higher levels of vitamin E

PRACTICE

Selegiline is a second-line therapy in Alzheimer disease.

Evidence

- **Source:** Birks J, Flicker L. Selegiline for Alzheimer's disease. *Cochrane Database Syst Rev.* 2000;(2):CD000442.
- **Takeaways:**
  - A meta-analysis demonstrated some benefit of selegiline in treating cognitive deficit but not enough to warrant consideration as first line therapy.
- **Notes:**
  - Selegiline is a monoamine oxidase inhibitor (MAOI). Caution patients on taking it with diets heavy in tyramine (aged cheese, wines).

PRACTICE

Rivastigmine is first-line therapy for Lewy body dementia.

Evidence

- **Source:** McKeith I, Del Ser T, Spano P, et al. Efficacy of rivastigmine in dementia with Lewy bodies: a randomised, double-blind, placebo-controlled international study. *Lancet.* 2000;356(9247):2031.
- **Takeaways:**
  - 30% improvement in hallucinations, delusions, and anxiety from baseline in at least twice as many patients taking rivastigmine compared with placebo
- **Notes:**
  - Dementia with Lewy bodies is differentiated from other neurodegenerative diseases by its predominance of vivid visual hallucinations and delusions prior to the onset of cognitive decline.

Multiple Sclerosis

PRACTICE

Optic neuritis is considered a clinically isolated syndrome (CIS) that represents increased risk for the development of MS.

Evidence

- **Source:** ONTT Trial. Optic Neuritis Study Group. The 5-year risk of MS after optic neuritis. Experience of the optic neuritis treatment trial. *Neurology.* 1997;49(5):1404.
- **Takeaways:**
  - Patients experiencing optic neuritis had a 30% 5-year risk of developing MS.
  - Five-year risk was highly correlated with the initial number of brain lesions on MRI.
  - Mild visual loss and lack of pain with optic neuritis were associated with a lower 5-year risk of MS.
- **Notes:**
  - Optic neuritis is typically unilateral in MS, reflecting the asymmetric nature of MS.

PRACTICE

IFNb-1b is an effective treatment for relapsing-remitting (RLRM) MS.

Evidence

- **Source:** The IFNB Multiple Sclerosis Study Group. Interferon beta-1b is effective in relapsing-remitting multiple sclerosis. I. Clinical results of a multicenter, randomized, double-blind, placebo-controlled trial. *Neurology.* 1993;43(4):655–61.
- **Takeaways:**
  - Significantly reduced relapse rates with IFNb (1.27 exacerbations in placebo vs. 0.84 in 8 MIU treatment arm)
- **Notes:**
  - IFNb functions by modulating the level of inflammatory players, particularly past the blood-brain barrier.

PRACTICE

IFNb-1a is an effective treatment for RLRM MS.

Evidence

- **Source:** PRISMS Trial. PRISMS (Prevention of Relapses and Disability by Interferon beta-1a Subcutaneously in Multiple Sclerosis) Study Group. Randomised double-blind placebo-controlled study of interferon beta-1a in relapsing/remitting multiple sclerosis. *Lancet.* 1999;353(9153):678.
- **Takeaways:**
  - Significantly lower relapse rate and disability with IFNb-1a at 1 and 2 years
  - Time to first relapse prolonged by 3 to 5 months depending on dosage
- **Notes:**
  - Because IFNb-1a is delivered via subcutaneous injections, skin reactions (including necrosis) are a common side effect.

PRACTICE

Glatiramer acetate is an effective treatment for RLRM MS.

Evidence

- **Source:** Johnson KP, Brooks BR, Cohen JA, et al. Copolymer 1 reduces relapse rate and improves disability in relapsing-remitting multiple sclerosis: results of a phase III multi-center, double-blind placebo-controlled trial. The Copolymer 1 Multiple Sclerosis Study Group. *Neurology.* 1995;45(7):1268–75.
- **Takeaways:**
  - 29% relative reduction in 2-year relapse rate with glatiramer compared with placebo
- **Notes:**
  - Glatiramer acts as a decoy of myelin basic protein.

PRACTICE

Fingolimod is an effective treatment for RLRM MS.

Evidence

- **Source:** FREEDOMS Trial. Kappos L, Radue EW, O'Connor P, et al,; FREEDOMS Study Group. A placebo-controlled trial of oral fingolimod in relapsing multiple sclerosis. *N Engl J Med.* 2010;362(5):387–401.
- **Takeaways:**
  - Significantly decreased 1-year relapse and disability rates
- **Source:** TRANSFORMS Trial. Cohen JA, Barkhof F, Comi G, et al.; TRANSFORMS Study Group. Oral fingolimod or intramuscular interferon for relapsing multiple sclerosis. *N Engl J Med.* 2010;362(5):402–15.
- **Takeaways:**
  - Compared with IFNb-1a, fingolimod was superior in reducing relapse rates.
- **Notes:**
  - Fingolimod was a breakthrough for MS therapy because it is administered by mouth rather than via injection, which many patients do not like.
  - Common adverse effects include mild transaminitis and atrioventricular block.

PRACTICE

Patients with MS should have adequate vitamin D supplementation as needed (e.g., Northern Hemisphere).

Evidence

- **Source:** Sintzel MB, Rametta M, Reder AT. Vitamin D and multiple sclerosis: a comprehensive review. *Neurol Ther.* 2018;7(1):59–85.
- **Takeaways:**
  - Increasing evidence from variety of studies, from observational to mendelian randomization, that suggest there is a causal association between vitamin D levels and risk of MS
- **Notes:**
  - Interestingly, the incidence of MS is higher in the Northern Hemisphere, where there is greater risk of vitamin D deficiency.

Peripheral Neuropathy

PRACTICE

Pregabalin is first-line treatment for painful diabetic neuropathy.

Evidence

- **Source:** Derry S, Bell RF, Straube S, et al. Pregabalin for neuropathic pain in adults. *Cochrane Database Syst Rev.* 2019;1(1):CD007076.
- **Takeaways:**
  - Significant (30%+) pain reduction with pregabalin for painful diabetic neuropathy
  - Did not demonstrate efficacy in central neuropathic pain
- **Notes:**
  - Common side effects include somnia, decreased concentration, and weight gain.
  - Different societies have differing recommendations on first-line therapies.

PRACTICE

Serotonin-norepinephrine reuptake inhibitors (SNRIs) such as duloxetine and venlafaxine are first-line treatment for pain due to diabetic neuropathy.

Evidence

- **Source:** Bril V, England J, Franklin GM, et al.; American Academy of Neurology; American Association of Neuromuscular and Electrodiagnostic Medicine; American Academy of Physical Medicine and Rehabilitation. Evidence-based guideline: treatment of painful diabetic neuropathy: report of the American Academy of Neurology, the American Association of Neuromuscular and Electrodiagnostic Medicine, and the American Academy of Physical Medicine and Rehabilitation. *Neurology.* 2011;76(20):1758–65.
- **Takeaways:**
  - Studies have suggested moderate (~20% more than placebo) pain relief with venlafaxine/ duloxetine.
- **Notes:**
  - SNRIs should not be combined with MAOIs.
  - SNRIs can potentiate warfarin via inhibition of P450.

PRACTICE

TCAs are first-line treatment for painful diabetic neuropathy.

Evidence

- **Source:** Max MB, Lynch SA, Muir J, et al. Effects of desipramine, amitriptyline, and fluoxetine on pain in diabetic neuropathy. *N Engl J Med.* 1992;326:1250–6.
- **Takeaways:**
  - TCAs were as effective or superior to fluoxetine and placebo for painful diabetic neuropathy.
- **Notes:**
  - TCAs should be used cautiously, if at all, in patients with cardiovascular disease.

PRACTICE

NSAIDs are not recommended for neuropathic pain management.

Evidence

- **Source:** Moore RA, Chi CC, Wiffen PJ, et al. Oral nonsteroidal anti-inflammatory drugs for neuropathic pain. *Cochrane Database Syst Rev.* 2015;10:CD010902.

- **Takeaways:**
  - No significant pain reduction from NSAID use in peripheral neuropathy
- **Notes:**
  - NSAIDs control pain via inhibition of prostaglandins, so this makes mechanistic sense why neuropathic pain would not be amenable to NSAID treatment.

PRACTICE

Early glucocorticoid therapy is recommended for maximizing facial nerve function recovery.

Evidence

- **Source:** de Almeida JR, Al Khabori M, Guyatt GH, et al. Combined corticosteroid and antiviral treatment for Bell palsy: a systematic review and meta-analysis. *JAMA.* 2009;302(9):985–93.
- **Takeaways:**
  - Relative risk 0.69 (confidence interval 0.55 to 0.87) for facial nerve dysfunction with glucocorticoid therapy; number needed to treat = 11
  - Relative risk 0.54 when glucocorticoids and antivirals combined
  - No significant change in outcomes with antivirals alone
- **Notes:**
  - Early glucocorticoid therapy is often accompanied by antiviral therapy (e.g., acyclovir).

Other Neurology

PRACTICE

Riluzole is initiated upon amyotrophic lateral sclerosis diagnosis to slow the progression of disease and for a potentially small reduction in mortality.

Evidence

- **Source:** Bensimon G, Lacomblez L, Meininger V. A controlled trial of riluzole in amyotrophic lateral sclerosis. ALS/Riluzole Study Group. *N Engl J Med* 1994;330(9):585.
- **Takeaways:**
  - Significant mortality benefit at 12 months in patients on riluzole
    - 19% mortality benefit overall
    - 38% mortality benefit for bulbar-onset disease
    - 10% mortality benefit for limb-onset disease
- **Source:** Lacomblez L, Bensimon G, Leigh PN, et al. Dose-ranging study of riluzole in amyotrophic lateral sclerosis. Amyotrophic Lateral Sclerosis/Riluzole Study Group II. *Lancet.* 1996;347(9013):1425.
- **Takeaways:**
  - 6.2% mortality benefit at 18 months
- **Notes:**
  - Riluzole is an antiglutamate agent.

PRACTICE

SBP is lowered to a goal of less than 140 during acute intracranial hemorrhage.

Evidence

- **Source:** INTERACT Trial. Anderson CS, Huang Y, Wang JG, et al.; INTERACT Investigators. Intensive blood pressure reduction in acute cerebral haemorrhage trial (INTERACT): a randomised pilot trial. *Lancet Neurol.* 2008;7(5):391–9.
- **Takeaways:**
  - 22.6% less intracranial hematoma growth with intensive blood pressure control
  - Intensive blood pressure lowering was well-tolerated.
- **Source:** INTERACT-2 Trial. Anderson CS, Heeley E, Huang Y, et al.; INTERACT2 Investigators. Rapid blood-pressure lowering in patients with acute intracerebral hemorrhage. *N Engl J Med.* 2013;368(25):2355–65.
- **Takeaways:**
  - Although intensive blood pressure control did not improve mortality or severe disability (barely missed significance at $P = .06$), it did improve functional outcomes (0.87 OR for greater disability), suggesting that intensive control is likely beneficial.
- **Source:** ATACH Investigators. Antihypertensive treatment of acute cerebral hemorrhage. *Crit Care Med.* 2010 Feb;38(2):637–48.
- **Takeaways:**
  - No difference in mortality in patients who received intensive blood pressure control versus standard control
- **Notes:**
  - A newer trial known as INTERACT 2 found opposing results with the aforementioned studies, but it is likely that this is due to its study design (blood pressure control only for 1 day versus 7 days; antihypertensive freedom of choice).

Nephrology

Acute Kidney Injury

PRACTICE

Fractional excretion of sodium (FENa) is often used to determine whether an acute kidney injury (AKI) is due to prerenal, intrarenal, or postrenal etiologies.

Evidence

- **Source:** Espinel CH. The FENa test. Use in the differential diagnosis of acute renal failure. *JAMA*. 1976;236(6):579–81.
- **Takeaways:**
  - Patients with prerenal azotemia had a FENa less than 1%.
  - Patients with acute tubular necrosis (ATN) had a FENa greater than 3%.
- **Notes:**
  - Based on setting, the cutoff FENa for ATN can vary between greater than 2% and greater than 4%. In general, FENa greater than 2% is considered another piece of evidence for ATN.
  - Do not use in the following scenarios or comorbidities:
    - Significant chronic kidney disease (CKD)
    - Active diuretic use (use fractional excretion of urea [FEUrea] instead)
    - Nonoliguric patients

PRACTICE

FEUrea is used to determine whether an AKI is due to prerenal, intrarenal, or postrenal etiologies when a patient is actively on diuretics.

EVIDENCE

- **Source:** Kaplan AA, Kohn OF. Fractional excretion of urea as a guide to renal dysfunction. *Am J Nephrol.* 1992;12(1–2):49–54.
- **Takeaways:**
  - Despite loop diuretic usage, FEUrea less than 35% was sensitive for predicting prerenal AKI.
- **Source:** Carvouncis CP, Nisar S, Guro-Razuman S. Significance of the fractional excretion of urea in the differential diagnosis of acute renal failure. *Kidney Int.* 2002;62(6):2223–9.
- **Takeaways:**
  - In diuretic use, FEUrea less than 35% was superior to FENa in differentiating between prerenal AKI and ATN.
- **Notes:**
  - FEUrea greater than 50% is used as a predictor of intrinsic renal damage.

PRACTICE

During AKI, nephrotoxins are avoided. These most prominently include NSAIDs, PPIs, ACE inhibitors (ACEIs)/angiotensin receptor blockers (ARBs), fenofibrates, and bowel preps (primarily sodium phosphate).

Evidence

- **Source:** Patrono C, Dunn MJ. The clinical significance of inhibition of renal prostaglandin synthesis. *Kidney Int.* 1987;32:1–12.
- **Source:** Yang Y, George KC, Shang WF, et al. Proton-pump inhibitors use, and risk of acute kidney injury: a meta-analysis of observational studies. *Drug Des Devel Ther.* 2017;11:1291–9.
- **Source:** Brar S, Ye F, James MT, et al.; Interdisciplinary Chronic Disease Collaboration. Association of angiotensin-converting enzyme inhibitor or angiotensin receptor blocker use with outcomes after acute kidney injury. *JAMA Intern Med.* 2018;178(12):1681–1690.
- **Source:** Layton JB, Klemmer PJ, Christiansen CF, et al. Sodium phosphate does not increase risk for acute kidney injury after routine colonoscopy, compared with polyethylene glycol. *Clin Gastroenterol Hepatol.* 2014;12:1514–21.
- **Takeaways:**
  - NSAIDs inhibit the native vasodilatory effects of renal prostaglandin on the renal arterioles, decreasing renal blood flow.
  - Meta-analysis of PPI use in more than 2 million patients yielded pooled adjusted relative risk of 1.61 for risk of AKI with PPI use.
  - ACEI/ARB use during AKI is associated with higher risk of hospitalization for a renal cause but lower mortality at 2 years.
  - No association of ACEI/ARB use during AKI and progression to end-stage renal disease (ESRD)
  - AKI rates were similar for oral sodium phosphate and polyethylene glycol bowel prep.
- **Notes:**
  - There are some conflicting data on ACEI/ARB use during AKI, but current clinical practice is to hold ACEI/ARB because the long-term benefits of ACEI/ARBs likely do not cease with holding of the medications for the duration of an episode of AKI.
  - The principal concern with bowel preps is dehydration and augmentation of a prerenal AKI. Some agents (e.g., phosphate containing preparations) can deposit within renal parenchyma. Osmotic preparations are the safest.

PRACTICE

Periprocedure hydration remains the single most important prophylactic measure for prevention of contrast-induced nephropathy (CIN).

Evidence

- **Source:** Reinecke H, Fobker M, Wellmann J, et al. A randomized controlled trial comparing hydration therapy to additional hemodialysis or N-acetylcysteine for the prevention of contrast medium-induced nephropathy: the Dialysis-versus-Diuresis (DVD) Trial. *Clin Res Cardiol.* 2007;96(3):130–9.
- **Takeaways:**
  - No significant difference in rates of CIN in prehydration versus N-acetylcysteine administration groups prior to administration of a significant contrast load
- **Notes:**
  - Evidence for effectiveness of interventions such as N-acetylcysteine or sodium bicarbonate is currently lacking.
  - If your patient has an elevated creatinine and you intend to order an intervention that involves contrast, contact your radiology department—they have guidelines for how much prehydration is indicated prior to these interventions.

PRACTICE

Metformin is used with careful monitoring in patients with CKD, due to risk of lactic acidosis.

Evidence

- **Source:** Lazarus B, Wu A, Shin JI, et al. Association of metformin use with risk of lactic acidosis across the range of kidney function: a community-based cohort study. *JAMA Intern Med.* 2018;178(7):903–10.
- **Takeaways:**
  - No significant increase in lactic acidosis with metformin use at glomerular filtration rate (GFR) greater than 30
- **Source:** Inzucchi SE, Lipska KJ, Mayo H, et al. Metformin in patients with type 2 diabetes and kidney disease: a systematic review. *JAMA.* 2014;312(24):2668–75.
- **Takeaways:**
  - Excellent systematic review of 818 studies (65 meeting inclusion criteria), which found limited evidence of lactic acidosis with metformin use in CKD (GFR >30)
- **Notes:**
  - Although metformin use in CKD has been an area of conflicting evidence, more of the recent evidence has favored cautious use with close monitoring, particularly in GFR greater than 30.

PRACTICE

In an AKI, metformin is held due to increased risk for lactic acidosis and nephrotoxicity.

Evidence

- **Source:** Connelly PJ, Lonergan M, Soto-Pedre E, et al. Acute kidney injury, plasma lactate concentrations and lactic acidosis in metformin users: a GoDarts study. *Diabetes Obes Metab.* 2017;19(11):1579–86.

- **Takeaways:**
  - Lactic acidosis more likely in patients on metformin with AKI
  - Likelihood of lactic acidosis increased with severity of AKI
- **Notes:**
  - Although there is no firm guideline on this topic due to the lack of definitive evidence, the expert recommendation is to withhold metformin during significant AKI and exercise clinical judgment for less severe AKIs.

PRACTICE

Glucocorticoids should be used for suspected acute interstitial nephritis.

Evidence

- **Source:** Galpin JE, Shinaberger JH, Stanley TM, et al. Acute interstitial nephritis due to methicillin. *Am J Med.* 1978;65(5):756–65.
- **Takeaways:**
  - Remission of acute interstitial nephritis (AIN) is quicker with steroid administration.
- **Source:** Ramachandran R, Kumar K, Nada R, et al. Drug-induced acute interstitial nephritis: a clinicopathological study and comparative trial of steroid regimens. *Indian J Nephrol.* 2015;25(5):281–6.
- **Takeaways:**
  - Type of steroid administration (oral vs. pulse) is equivalent in achieving remission of AIN.
- **Notes:**
  - The offending drug(s) should be promptly discontinued when AIN is suspected.
  - Common drugs causing AIN can be remembered by the mnemonic PND-SR:
    - **P**enicillins (including cephalosporins)/Pembrolizumab
    - **N**SAIDs
    - **D**iuretics
    - **S**ulfonamides
    - **R**ifampin

PRACTICE

In noncritically ill patients, there is no significant difference in outcomes when using balanced crystalloids or saline for fluid management.

Evidence

- **Source:** SALT-ED Trial. Self WH, Semler MW, Wanderer JP, et al.; SALT-ED Investigators. Balanced crystalloids versus saline in noncritically ill adults. *N Engl J Med.* 2018;378:819–828.
- **Takeaways:**
  - No difference in hospital-free days between balanced crystalloids and saline use in noncritically ill patients
  - Study conducted in emergency department setting
- **Notes:**
  - Normal Plasma Concentrations:
    - Na^+ 135 to 145
    - Cl^- 100 to 110

- K^+ 3.5 to 5.0
- HCO_3^- 22 to 26
- 280 to 295 mOsm/L
- Lactated Ringer Composition:
  - Na^+ 130
  - Cl^- 109
  - K^+ 4.0
  - Ca^{2+} 3.0
  - HCO_3^- 28
  - Lactate 28 to 29 mEq
  - 273 mOsm/L
- Normal Saline Composition:
  - Na^+ 154
  - Cl^- 154
  - 308 mOsm/L

PRACTICE

In critically ill patients, balanced crystalloids such as lactated Ringer are preferred over saline.

Evidence

- **Source:** SMART Trial. Semler MW, Self WH, Wanderer JP, et al.; SMART Investigators and the Pragmatic Critical Care Research Group. Balanced crystalloids versus saline in critically ill adults. *N Engl J Med.* 2018;378:829–39.
- **Takeaways:**
  - Reduced mortality (10.3% vs. 11.1%) with use of balanced crystalloids versus saline in critically ill patients
  - Marginally lower rate of new renal-replacement therapy (2.5% vs. 2.9%) or permanent renal dysfunction (6.4% vs. 6.6%) with use of balanced crystalloids
  - Study conducted in ICU setting
- **Notes:**
  - Lactated Ringer is also known as Hartmann solution.
  - Lactated Ringer was originally developed without the lactate, and lactate was added later for buffering purposes.

PRACTICE

In ATN, renal replacement therapy (RRT) is initiated when a clear need for hemodialysis is apparent (e.g., severe metabolic derangements, oliguria with profound volume overload).

Evidence

- **Source:** ATN Trial. VA/NIH Acute Renal Failure Trial Network; Palevsky PM, Zhang JH, O'Connor TZ, et al. Intensity of renal support in critically ill patients with acute kidney injury. *N Engl J Med.* 2008;359(1):7–20.
- **Takeaways:**
  - No improvement in mortality with more intensive RRT
- **Notes:**
  - Intensive RRT = 6× per week, continuous venovenous hemodiafiltration (CVVHDF) at 35 mL/kg/h
  - Less-intense RRT = 3× per week, CVVHDF at 20 mL/kg/h

PRACTICE

In patients with AKI and septic shock, RRT should be delayed in critically ill patients with AKI but no urgent indication for hemodialysis (e.g., severe metabolic derangements, oliguria with profound volume overload).

Evidence

- **Source:** IDEAL-ICU Trial. Barbar SD, Clere-Jehl R, Bourredjem A, et al.; IDEAL-ICU Trial Investigators and the CRICS TRIGGERSEP Network. Timing of renal-replacement therapy in patients with acute kidney injury and sepsis. *N Engl J Med.* 2018;379(15):1431–42.
- **Takeaways:**
  - No difference in 90-day mortality between early and delayed RRT initiation in ICU patients with AKI and septic shock
  - Lower RRT use in delayed-initiation arm
- **Source:** GroupAKIKI Trial. Gaudry S, Hajage D, Schortgen F, et al.; AKIKI Study Group. Initiation strategies for renal-replacement therapy in the intensive care unit. *N Engl J Med.* 2016;375(2):122–33.
- **Takeaways:**
  - No mortality difference between early versus late RRT in ICU patients with AKI
- **Notes:**
  - Evidence is not clear cut but suggests that delayed initiation is better because there is no benefit to early initiation.

Cardiorenal Syndrome

PRACTICE

In acutely decompensated heart failure, diuretics may be administered in either bolus or by continuous infusion.

Evidence

- **Source:** DOSE Trial. Felker GM, Lee KL, Bull DA, et al.; NHLBI Heart Failure Clinical Research Network. Diuretic strategies in patients with acute decompensated heart failure. *N Engl J Med.* 2011;364(9):797–805.
- **Takeaways:**
  - Bolus and continuous diuretic infusions are equivalent for symptomatic improvement in acutely decompensated heart failure.
  - Faster symptomatic improvement with high-dose diuresis compared with low dosage
- **Notes:**
  - Most commonly, bolus dosing is used. Per current American Heart Association (AHA) guidelines, continuous intravenous (IV) diuresis is recommended only as step-up therapy for patients who remain refractory to bolus diuresis.

PRACTICE

In the setting of cardiorenal syndrome, dopamine and low-dose nesiritide are not efficacious adjuncts to traditional diuresis.

Evidence

- **Source:** ROSE Trial. Chen HH, Anstrom KJ, Givertz MM, et al.; NHLBI Heart Failure Clinical Research Network. Low-dose dopamine or low-dose nesiritide in acute heart failure with renal dysfunction: the ROSE acute heart failure randomized trial. *JAMA*. 2013;310(23):2533–43.

- **Takeaways:**
  - In cardiorenal syndrome, dopamine or nesiritide in adjunct to diuretics did not improve congestion, renal function, or clinical outcomes.
- **Notes:**
  - In theory, dopamine and nesiritide would increase forward flow into the kidneys, thereby acting synergistically with diuretics (more delivery to the respective sites of action i.e., transporters).

PRACTICE

In heart failure exacerbation refractory to diuresis, ultrafiltration is an alternative means of removing fluid.

Evidence

- **Source:** CARRESS-HF Trial. Bart BA, Goldsmith SR, Lee KL, et al.; Heart Failure Clinical Research Network. Ultrafiltration in decompensated heart failure with cardiorenal syndrome. *N Engl J Med*. 2012;367(24):2296–304.
- **RCT**
- **Takeaways:**
  - No difference in symptomatic improvement or weight loss between ultrafiltration and pharmacologic diuresis
  - Ultrafiltration worse than pharmacologic diuresis for renal function
  - Ultrafiltration associated with higher rate of adverse events
- **Notes:**
  - Ultrafiltration is reserved as a last resort for patients refractory to pharmacologic diuresis.
  - These results are contradictory to an earlier trial, UNLOAD. However, expert consensus is that CARRESS-HF is more likely accurate given more rigid, appropriate methodology and protocols.

Hyponatremia

PRACTICE

In the setting of hyperglycemia, pseudohyponatremia occurs and is corrected using a factor of 1.6 or 2.4 mEq/L per 100 mg/dL additional blood glucose.

Evidence

- **Source**: Katz MA. Hyperglycemia-induced hyponatremia—calculation of expected serum sodium depression. *N Engl J Med*. 1973;289(16):843–4.
- **Takeaways:**
  - 1.6 mEq/L decline in sodium per 100 mg/dL blood glucose units greater than 100 mg/dL
  - This correction factor is based on modeling rather than actual patient data.
- **Source**: Hillier TA, Abbott RD, Barrett EJ. Hyponatremia: evaluating the correction factor for hyperglycemia. *Am J Med*. 1999;106(4):399–403.
- **Takeaways:**
  - Correction factor of –2.4 mEq/L deemed to be more accurate than the –1.6 mEq/L factor by Katz in 1973
  - Actual patient plasma sodium levels measured

- **Notes:**
  - The correction factor used is variable between institutions and individual clinicians. Based on the study type and rigor, -2.4 mEq/L is likely the better correction factor.
  - Hyponatremia is caused by extracellular hyperosmolality, causing a shift of water out of cells, leading to a dilution of plasma sodium levels.

PRACTICE

Chronic hyponatremia is corrected to a maximum of 4 to 6 mEq/L per 24 hours.

Evidence

- **Source**: Adrogue HJ, Madias NE. Hyponatremia. *N Engl J Med*. 2000;342(21):1581–9.
- Review article
- **Takeaways:**
  - The majority of osmotic demyelination syndrome occurred when hyponatremia was corrected by greater than 12 mEq/L/day.
- **Notes:**
  - Based on the increased risk threshold of 12 mEq/L/day in the aforementioned review, expert consensus has been to maximally correct by 4 to 6 mEq/L/day.
  - Acute hyponatremia is defined as hyponatremia occurring within 48 hours. To qualify, the patient must have had a recorded normal sodium level and then an acutely recorded drop in sodium.
  - Acute hyponatremia has no correction limit because there has not been enough time for equilibration to occur between intra/extracellular compartments.

PRACTICE

In the setting of acute neurologic symptoms, severe hyponatremia should be treated with hypertonic saline (100 cc).

Evidence

- **Source:** Spasovski G, Vanholder R, Allolio B, et al.; Hyponatraemia Guideline Development Group. Clinical practice guideline on diagnosis and treatment of hyponatraemia. *Eur J Endocrinol*. 2014;170(3):G1–47.
- **Takeaways:**
  - From analysis of multiple small studies, it was deemed that among currently available options, 3% saline provides a reasonably quick correction of hyponatremia and symptomatic improvement.
- **Notes:**
  - If patient continues to be symptomatic, administer up to two boluses of 100 cc hypertonic saline.
  - Sodium levels should be checked routinely, including approximately 20 minutes after administration of a hypertonic bolus.

PRACTICE

dDAVP (desmopressin) "clamping" can be used to prevent overcorrection of hyponatremia, particularly in severe cases or cases with increased risk for overcorrection.

Evidence

- **Source**: Perianayagam A, Sterns RH, Silver SM, et al. dDAVP is effective in preventing and reversing inadvertent overcorrection of hyponatremia. *Clin J Am Soc Nephrol.* 2008;3(2):331–6.
- **Source**: MacMillan TE, Cavalcanti RB. Outcomes in severe hyponatremia treated with and without desmopressin. *Am J Med.* 2018;131(3):317.e1–317.e10.
- **Source:** Retrospective observational study
- **Takeaways:**
  - dDAVP clamping virtually guarantees that sodium levels will not overcorrect.
  - dDAVP clamping is not associated with greater adverse events.
  - Hospital stay was, on average, 1 day greater with dDAVP clamping.
- **Notes:**
  - dDAVP clamping means iatrogenically inducing syndrome of inappropriate antidiuretic hormone to prevent overcorrection of hyponatremia by administering exogenous antidiuretic hormone (i.e., dDAVP).
  - dDAVP clamping is convenient because it requires no monitoring of sodium levels while the dDAVP is active.
  - Risk factors for overcorrection of hyponatremia include:
    - Malnutrition
    - Active thiazide diuretic use
    - Hypovolemia
    - Severe hyponatremia

Hypernatremia

PRACTICE

Chronic hypernatremia is typically corrected no faster than 12 mEq/L/day to decrease the theoretical risk of cerebral edema and seizures.

Evidence

- **Source**: Chauhan K, Pattharanitima P, Patel N,et al. Rate of correction of hypernatremia and health outcomes in critically ill patients. *Clin J Am Soc Nephrol.* 2019;14(5):656–63.
- **Takeaways:**
  - No increased mortality or risk of adverse events with rapid correction of hypernatremia (>12 mEq/L/day)
- **Notes:**
  - Typical goal correction rate is 10 mEq/L/day given the theoretically increased risk threshold of 12 mEq/L/day.
  - Acute hypernatremia correction has no limits given lack of time for significant equilibration of intra/extracellular compartments.

Hypokalemia

PRACTICE

Magnesium should be repleted if low to facilitate correction of hypokalemia.

Evidence

- **Source:** Huang C-H, Kuo E. Mechanism of hypokalemia in magnesium deficiency. *J Am Soc Nephrol.* 2007;18(10):2649–52.
- Review article

- **Takeaways:**
  - Hypomagnesemia may increase distal potassium section and thus contribute to resistant hypokalemia.
- **Notes:**
  - Magnesium inhibits renal outer medullary potassium channels, thereby leading to increased potassium secretion.

Hyperkalemia

PRACTICE

IV calcium is administered immediately in severe hyperkalemia to stabilize the myocardium.

Evidence

- **Source:** Winkler AW, Hoff HE, Smith PK. Factors affecting the toxicity of potassium. *Am J Physiol.* 1939;127:430.
- **Takeaways:**
  - Calcium directly antagonizes the effect of potassium on cardiomyocyte membranes.
  - Physiology experiments conducted on dogs
- **Notes:**
  - Calcium should alleviate hyperkalemia-induced ECG changes within 3 to 5 minutes. If no change is seen, administer further calcium gluconate.
  - Be careful of administering calcium if the patient is on digoxin (can potentiate)!
  - Calcium gluconate is preferred to calcium chloride due to decreased risk of tissue necrosis if extravasated.

Hypocalcemia

PRACTICE

Serum calcium levels need to be considered in conjunction with serum albumin levels.

Evidence

- **Source:** Payne RB, Little AJ, Williams RB, Milner JR. Interpretation of serum calcium in patients with abnormal serum proteins. *Br Med J.* 1973;4(5893):643–6.
- **Takeaways:**
  - For every 1 g/dL of hypoalbuminemia, the true (total) serum calcium level is corrected by approximately +0.8 mEq/L.
- **Notes:**
  - Free (ionized) calcium is the physiologically active form.
  - Serum calcium (reported on routine labs) is mostly bound to albumin.
  - Hypoalbuminemia can lead to pseudohypocalcemia (falsely low serum calcium level since it is mostly bound to albumin).
  - Albumin levels do NOT affect free (ionized) calcium levels.

PRACTICE

Large amounts of citrate (regional anticoagulation in RRT, massive infusion of blood products) should be avoided or used only with careful monitoring in patients with poor liver synthetic function due to risk of hypocalcemia.

Evidence

- **Source:** Link A, Klingele M, Speer T, et al. Total-to-ionized calcium ratio predicts mortality in continuous renal replacement therapy with citrate anticoagulation in critically ill patients. *Crit Care.* 2012;16(3):R97.
- **Source:** Zhang W, Bai M, Yu Y, et al. Safety and efficacy of regional citrate anticoagulation for continuous renal replacement therapy in liver failure patients: a systematic review and meta-analysis. *Crit Care.* 2019;23(1):22.
- **Takeaways:**
  - 33.5 times greater risk of mortality in continuous renal replacement therapy (CRRT) with regional citrate anticoagulation administration in critically ill patients with AKI
  - More recent meta-analysis showed no significant difference in pH, lactate, or total/free Ca^{2+} ratio in patients with liver failure on CRRT with citrate anticoagulation.
- **Notes**
  - Most sensitive marker of citrate accumulation is ionized hypocalcemia.

PRACTICE

Hypocalcemia is treated prior to treatment of acidosis to ensure that the physiologically active free calcium does not fall further.

Evidence

- **Source:** Cooper MS, Gittoes NJL. Diagnosis and management of hypocalcaemia. *BMJ.* 2008;336(7656):1298–302.
- **Takeaways:**
  - Treat hypocalcemia prior to treating acidosis.
- **Notes:**
  - In major shifts of pH, measure the free ionized calcium to check for true hypocalcemia.
  - Acidosis leads to decreased binding of calcium to albumin (thus low measured serum calcium which is bound to albumin) and increased free ionized calcium.
  - Alkalosis leads to increased calcium binding by albumin and decreased free ionized calcium.
  - Do not mix or administer calcium and sodium bicarbonate through the same line! This can lead to calcium precipitation.

Chronic Kidney Disease

PRACTICE

The Cockcroft-Gault equation was the first widely accepted formula for estimating GFR.

Evidence

- **Source:** Cockcroft, DW, Gault MH. Prediction of creatinine clearance from serum creatinine. *Nephron.* 1976;16(1):31–41.
- **Takeaways:**
  - The Cockcroft-Gault equation was derived from 249 patients.
  - Cockcroft-Gault variables include sex, age, weight, height, and serum creatinine.
- **Notes:**
  - Cockcroft-Gault overestimates true GFR.

PRACTICE

The Modification of Diet in Renal Disease (MDRD) equation is another more recent equation used to estimate GFR.

Evidence

- **Source:** Levey AS, Bosch JP, Lewis JB, et al. A more accurate method to estimate glomerular filtration rate from serum creatinine: a new prediction equation. Modification of Diet in Renal Disease Study Group. *Ann Intern Med.* 1999;130(6):461–70.
- **Takeaways:**
  - The MDRD equation was derived from more than 1000 patients in an effort to simplify the prediction of GFR.
  - MDRD variables include sex, race, age, and serum creatinine.
- **Source:** Levey AS, Coresh J, Greene T, et al.; Chronic Kidney Disease Epidemiology Collaboration. Using standardized serum creatinine values in the modification of diet in renal disease study equation for estimating glomerular filtration rate. *Ann Int Med.* 2006;145(4):247–54.
- **Takeaways:**
  - MDRD equation outperformed the Cockcroft-Gault equation in accuracy.
- **Notes:**
  - MDRD underestimates GFR when greater than 60.

PRACTICE

The CKD-EPI equation is now one of the commonly used equations to estimate GFR.

Evidence

- **Source:** Levey AS, Stevens LA, Schmid CH, et al.; CKD-EPI (Chronic Kidney Disease Epidemiology Collaboration). A new equation to estimate glomerular filtration rate. *Ann Intern Med.* 2009;150(9):604–12.
- **Takeaways:**
  - The CKD-EPI equation was derived from a linear regression of more than 8000 patients.
  - CKD-EPI variables include serum creatinine, sex, race, and age.
- **Source:** Inker LA, Schmid CH, Tighiouart H, et al.; CKD-EPI Investigators. Estimating glomerular filtration rate from serum creatinine and cystatin C. *N Engl J Med.* 2012;367(1):20–9.
- **Takeaways:**
  - CKD-EPI equation outperformed the MDRD equation in predicting GFR and in sensitivity of GFR less than 60.
- **Notes:**
  - Works well for higher GFR (>60), thus preferred for routine use throughout the hospital

PRACTICE

Vascular access for predialysis patients is typically initiated during stage 4 CKD to prepare for the inevitable complete loss of kidney function.

Evidence

- **Source:** Hod T, Patibandla BK, Vin Y, et al. Arteriovenous fistula placement in the elderly: when is the optimal time? *J Am Soc Nephrol.* 2015;26(2):448–56.

- **Takeaways:**
  - Placement of an arteriovenous fistula (AVF) greater than 6 to 9 months predialysis was not correlated with better success rates of dialysis using AVF.
  - For AVFs placed early, increased interventions were required to maintain AVF patency prior to dialysis start.
- **Source:** Woo K, Lok CE. New insights into dialysis vascular access: what is the optimal vascular access type and timing of access creation in CKD and dialysis patients? *Clin J Am Soc Nephrol.* 2016;11(8):1487–94.
- **Takeaways:**
  - Approximately 10% of patients do not begin dialysis for more than 2 years after reaching stage 4 CKD.
  - Unclear overall evidence surrounding the ideal time for initiating vascular access
- **Notes:**
  - Determination of the ideal time for obtaining vascular access depends on many factors, including race and gender, and should be undertaken with clinical judgment specific to each patient's case.

PRACTICE

ACEIs are routinely prescribed to slow the progression of CKD in diabetic patients with microalbuminuria.

Evidence

- **Source:** ACE Inhibitors in Diabetic Nephropathy Trialist Group. Should all patients with type 1 diabetes and microalbuminuria receive angiotensin-converting enzyme inhibitors? A meta-analysis of individual patient data. *Ann Intern Med.* 2001;134(5):370–9.
- Meta-analysis of 10 small RCTs
- **Takeaways:**
  - Increased likelihood of reverting to nonalbuminuric state
  - Significantly lower risk of progression to macroalbuminuria
- **Source:** Sano T, Hotta N, Kawamura T, et al. Effects of long-term enalapril treatment on persistent microalbuminuria in normotensive type 2 diabetic patients: results of a 4-year, prospective, randomized study. *Diabet Med.* 1996;13(2):120–4.
- RCT
- **Takeaways:**
  - ACEI group had decreased albuminuria over 48 months, whereas placebo group saw progression of albuminuria.
  - No change in creatinine clearance or blood pressure in control or intervention groups
- **Notes:**
  - ACEIs should be initiated as soon as microalbuminuria is confirmed. Do not delay!
  - ACEIs should be initiated carefully in diabetic nephropathy because there may be a temporary acute decline in GFR and hyperkalemia (due to compounding effect of ACEIs on type 4 renal tubular acidosis [hyporeninemic hypoaldosteronism] also seen in advanced diabetic nephropathy).

PRACTICE

ACEIs are routinely prescribed to slow the progression of CKD in nondiabetic patients with CKD, regardless of etiology.

Evidence

- **Source:** Gansevoort RT, Sluiter WJ, Hemmelder MH, et al. Antiproteinuric effect of blood-pressure-lowering agents: a meta-analysis of comparative trials. *Nephrol Dial Transplant.* 1995;10(11):1963–74.
- **Takeaways:**
  - ACEIs had a significantly greater antiproteinuric effect than other classes of antihypertensives.
  - All non-ACEI antihypertensives demonstrated a similarly low antiproteinuric effect dependent on the blood pressure reduction achieved.
- **Notes:**
  - The two most common causes of CKD are diabetes and hypertension.

PRACTICE

ARBs are equally as effective as reducing proteinuria in CKD as are ACEIs.

Evidence

- **Source:** Kunz R, Friedrich C, Wolbers M, Mann JFE. Meta-analysis: effect of monotherapy and combination therapy with inhibitors of the renin angiotensin system on proteinuria in renal disease. *Ann Intern Med.* 2008;148(1):30–48.
- **Takeaways:**
  - ARBs have similar antiproteinuric efficacy as ACEIs.
  - ACEIs and ARBs had a synergistic antiproteinuric effect greater than either alone.
- **Notes:**
  - If a patient is unable to tolerate ACEIs due to cough or angioedema, ARBs may be an alternative (refer to ONTARGET trial).

PRACTICE

Patients with CKD receive aggressive blood pressure control with goal blood pressure 130/80.

Evidence

- **Source:** Jafar TH, Stark PC, Schmid CH, et al.; AIPRD Study Group. Progression of chronic kidney disease: the role of blood pressure control, proteinuria, and angiotensin-converting enzyme inhibition: a patient-level meta-analysis. *Ann Intern Med.* 2003;139(4):244–52.
- Meta-analysis
- **Takeaways:**
  - Systolic blood pressure (SBP) of 110 to 129 may reduce CKD progression.
- **Source:** Anderson AH, Yang W, Townsend RR, et al.; Chronic Renal Insufficiency Cohort Study Investigators. Time-updated systolic blood pressure and the progression of chronic kidney disease: a cohort study. *Ann Intern Med.* 2015;162(4):258–65.
- Cohort study
- **Takeaways:**
  - SBP greater than 130 was associated with increased CKD progression.
- **Notes:**
  - The 2018 SPRINT trial began to popularize the goal of 130/80 for CKD patients, particularly to slow CKD progression, although the primary aim of the study was to examine cardiovascular outcomes by blood pressure control stringency.

PRACTICE

Daily sodium bicarbonate slows progression of CKD.

Evidence

- **Source:** AASK Trial. Raphael KL, Wei G, Baird BC, et al. Higher serum bicarbonate levels within the normal range are associated with better survival and renal outcomes in African Americans. *Kidney Int.* 2011;79(3):356.
- **Takeaways**
  - Higher serum bicarbonate was associated with decreased mortality, dialysis, and CKD progression.
- **Source:** Dobre M, Yang W, Chen J, et al.; CRIC Investigators. Association of serum bicarbonate with risk of renal and cardiovascular outcomes in CKD: a report from the Chronic Renal Insufficiency Cohort (CRIC) study. *Am J Kidney Dis.* 2013;62(4):670.
- **Takeaways:**
  - Lower bicarbonate levels were associated (3% higher per 1 mEq/L decrease) with increased CKD progression.

PRACTICE

Sodium glucose cotransporter-2 (SGLT2) inhibitors are used to decrease the progression of CKD.

Evidence

- **Source:** CREDENCE Trial. Perkovic V, Jardine MJ, Neal B, et al.; CREDENCE Trial Investigators. Canagliflozin and renal outcomes in type 2 diabetes and nephropathy. *N Engl J Med.* 2019;380:2295–306.
- Key inclusion criteria
  - GFR 30 to 90 mL/min
  - Albumin/Cr ratio 300 to 5000
  - All patients were on renin angiotensin aldosterone system (RAAS) agents.
- **Takeaways:**
  - Significantly lower risk (30% lower; 43.2% vs. 61.2%) of kidney failure with SGLT2 inhibitors (canagliflozin) compared with placebo
  - SGLT2 group also had significantly reduction in cardiovascular mortality and events.
- **Notes:**
  - SGLT2 inhibitors' key side effects:
    - Increased risk of UTIs
    - Increased risk for diabetic ketoacidosis (DKA)
    - Increased risk of lower limb amputation
    - Increased risk of Fournier gangrene

PRACTICE

Metabolic complications of CKD are typically screened following GFR thresholds.

Evidence

- **Source:** Moranne O, Froissart M, Rossert J, et al.; NephroTest Study Group. Timing of onset of CKD-related metabolic complications. *J Am Soc Nephrol.* 2009;20(1):164–71.

- **Takeaways:**
  - Anemia and hyperparathyroidism screening should start during early stage 3 CKD.
  - Hyperkalemia, hyperphosphatemia, and metabolic acidosis screening should start at GFR of 40 or less.
- **Notes:**
  - Screening practices vary widely by institution, but a general sense of when to pay attention to specific metabolic complications is useful.

PRACTICE

Dialysis initiation for patients with CKD stage 5 is based on symptoms, metabolic homeostasis, and tailored discussions with nephrologists. There is no set GFR threshold at which dialysis must be initiated.

Evidence

- **Source:** IDEAL Trial. Cooper BA, Branley P, Bulfone L, et al.; IDEAL Study. A randomized, controlled trial of early versus late initiation of dialysis. *N Engl J Med.* 2010;363(7):609–19.
- **Takeaways:**
  - No difference in mortality or clinical outcomes with early versus late dialysis initiation
- **Notes:**
  - Extremely low GFR (e.g., <10 mL/min/1.73m²) can be an indication for dialysis initiation regardless of symptomatology.

Primary Hypertension

PRACTICE

Per 2017 AHA ACC blood pressure guidelines, normal blood pressure is less than 120/80 with stage 1 hypertension beginning at 130/80. Thus the new blood pressure goal is less than 130/80, particularly for patients with CKD.

Evidence

- **Source:** SPRINT Trial. SPRINT Research Group; Wright JT Jr, Williamson JD, Whelton PK, et al. A randomized trial of intensive versus standard blood-pressure control. *N Engl J Med.* 2015;373(22):2103–16.
- **Takeaways:**
  - Intensive blood pressure control (<120 mm Hg SBP) showed a mortality benefit and improved cardiovascular outcomes compared with less intensive therapy (target <140 mm Hg).
  - Rates of AKI, orthostatic hypotension, and syncope increased.
- **Notes:**
  - Many providers have been hesitant to accept SPRINT trial results, and thus the shift toward a goal pressure of less than 130/80 has been slow and remains provider dependent.

PRACTICE

First-line antihypertensives include a thiazide, ACEI, or calcium channel blocker.

Evidence

- **Source:** ALLHAT Trial. The ALLHAT Officers and Coordinators for the ALLHAT Collaborative Research Group; Furberg CD, Wright JT Jr, Davis BR, et al. Major outcomes in high-risk hypertensive patients randomized to angiotensin-converting enzyme inhibitor or calcium channel blocker vs. diuretic: the Antihypertensive and Lipid-Lowering Treatment to Prevent Heart Attack Trial (ALLHAT). *JAMA.* 2002;288(23):2981–97.
- **Takeaways:**
  - No difference in cardiovascular events between chlorthalidone, amlodipine, and lisinopril
- **Notes:**
  - Although chlorthalidone was studied in this trial, hydrochlorothiazide is the most commonly prescribed thiazide antihypertensive.
    - Mainly phenomenon of cost and ease of access
    - Some evidence that hydrochlorothiazide does not have the same blood pressure– and cardiovascular event–lowering effects as chlorthalidone
  - Resistant hypertension is defined as blood pressure not meeting goal with three different classes of antihypertensives, at least one being a diuretic.

PRACTICE

The Dietary Approaches to Stop Hypertension (DASH) diet is the only proven diet that is recommended for improving hypertension.

Evidence

- **Source:** DASH Trial. Appel LJ, Moore TJ, Obarzanek E, et al. A clinical trial of the effects of dietary patterns on blood pressure. DASH Collaborative Research Group. *N Engl J Med.* 1997;336(16):1117–24.
- **Takeaways:**
  - DASH diet led to significant reduction in blood pressure for starting SBP less than 160 mm Hg.
- **Notes:**
  - DASH diet sodium limit: 2.3 g/day
  - DASH diet is rich in fruits, vegetables, low-fat dairy, grains, and lean meats.

Secondary Hypertension

PRACTICE

Renal artery stenosis is typically medically managed.

Evidence

- **Source:** CORAL Trial. Cooper CJ, Murphy TP, Cutlip DE, et al.; CORAL Investigators. Stenting and medical therapy for atherosclerotic renal-artery stenosis. *N Engl J Med.* 2014;370(1):13–22.
- **Takeaways:**
  - No improvement in either renal or cardiac outcomes with renal artery stenting in atherosclerotic renal artery stenosis
- **Notes:**
  - Stenting/angioplasty does provide an insignificant (–2 mm Hg) reduction in blood pressure compared with medical therapy.

Anemia

PRACTICE

High-dose IV iron may be considered in hemodialysis patients to reduce doses of erythropoiesis-stimulating agents or in refractory cases.

Evidence

- **Source:** PIVOTAL Trial. Macdougall IC, White C, Anker SD, et al.; PIVOTAL Investigators and Committees. Intravenous iron in patients undergoing maintenance hemodialysis. *N Engl J Med.* 2019;380:447–58.
- **Takeaways:**
  - Proactive, high-dose IV iron strategy resulted in lower doses of erythropoiesis-stimulating agent dosage requirements.
- **Notes:**
  - High-dose proactive iron strategy targets ferritin greater than 700.

PRACTICE

Use of erythropoiesis-stimulating agents in CKD should be considered at hemoglobin levels less than 9 g/dL and target hemoglobin levels of 10 to 11 g/dL, not higher.

Evidence

- **Source:** CHOIR Trial. Singh AK, Szczech L, Tang KL, et al.; CHOIR Investigators. Correction of anemia with epoetin alfa in chronic kidney disease. *N Engl J Med.* 2006;355(20):2085–98.
- **Source:** TREAT Trial. Pfeffer MA, Burdmann EA, Chen CY, et al.; TREAT Investigators. A trial of darbepoetin alfa in type 2 diabetes and chronic kidney disease. *N Engl J Med.* 2009;361(21):2019–32.
- **Takeaways:**
  - Both studies revealed increased mortality with higher hemoglobin goal (13 g/dL) for erythropoietin therapy.
- **Notes:**
  - Current recommendations are for a hemoglobin of 9 to 11 g/dL.

Glomerular Disease, Nephrotic

PRACTICE

Glucocorticoids are first-line therapy for minimal change disease (MCD).

Evidence

- **Source:** Black DA. Controlled trial of prednisone in adult patients with the nephrotic syndrome. *Br Med J.* 1970;3(5720):421–26.
- **Takeaways:**
  - Significant decrease in proteinuria of glucocorticoid administration in minimal change disease
  - Steroids did not have any significant long-term renal effects in any group.
- **Notes:**
  - MCD is a result of podocyte (foot process) effacement, leading to leakage of albumin into urine.

PRACTICE

Primary (idiopathic) membranous nephropathy is associated with antiphospholipase receptor A-2 antibody and is used as a serologic diagnostic aid.

Evidence

- **Source:** Beck LH, Bonegio RGB, Lambeau G, et al. M-type phospholipase A2 receptor as target antigen in idiopathic membranous nephropathy. *N Engl J Med.* 2009;361(1):11–21.
- **Takeaways:**
  - By Western blotting, 70% of patients with idiopathic membranous nephropathy were found to have antibodies to PLA2R.
- **Notes:**
  - PLA2R is found in normal podocytes.
  - Major secondary causes of membranous nephropathy include:
    - Penicillamine
    - Captopril
    - Malignancies
    - HBV/HCV

PRACTICE

The primary treatment for nonrapidly progressing membranous glomerulonephritis includes either rituximab or calcineurin inhibitors (lack of robust evidence).

Evidence

- **Source:** MENTOR Trial. Fervenza FC, Appel GB, Barbour SJ, et al.; MENTOR Investigators. Rituximab or cyclosporine in the treatment of membranous nephropathy. *N Engl J Med.* 2019;381(1):36–46.
- RCT
- **Takeaways:**
  - Rituximab was noninferior to cyclosporine at 12 months and superior at 24 months for treatment of membranous nephropathy (measured by remission of proteinuria).
- **Notes:**
  - Membranous nephropathy is the most common cause of nephrotic syndrome in adults.
  - For rapidly progressive membranoproliferative glomerulonephritis, patients should be immediately treated with steroids and cyclophosphamide.

Glomerular Disease, Nephritic

PRACTICE

Oral versus monthly IV cyclophosphamide regimens are equivocal and largely dependent on provider and patient preference.

Evidence

- **Source:** CYCLOPS Trial. De Groot K, Harper L, Jayne DRW, et al.; EUVAS (European Vasculitis Study Group). Pulse versus daily oral cyclophosphamide for induction of remission in antineutrophil cytoplasmic antibody-associated vasculitis: a randomized trial. *Ann of Intern Med.* 2009;150(10):670–80.

- **Takeaways:**
  - Pulse IV and oral regimens have equivalent rates and time to disease remission.
  - Lower relapse rate with oral dosing
  - Increased risk of leukopenia with oral dosing
- **Notes:**
  - Monthly IV dosing results in receipt of less overall cyclophosphamide.

PRACTICE

In patients with life- or organ-threatening ANCA-associated vasculitis, glucocorticoids are administered with either rituximab or cyclophosphamide.

Evidence

- **Source:** RAVE Trial. Stone JH, Merkel PA, Spiera R, et al.; RAVE-ITN Research Group. Rituximab versus cyclophosphamide for ANCA-associated vasculitis. *N Engl J Med.* 2010;363:221–32.
- **Source:** RITUXVAS Trial. Jones RB, Tervaert JWC, Hauser T, et al.; European Vasculitis Study Group. Rituximab versus cyclophosphamide in ANCA-associated renal vasculitis. *N Engl J Med.* 2010;363:211–20.
- **Takeaways:**
  - Rituximab therapy was noninferior to cyclophosphamide in ANCA-associated vasculitis, including renal vasculitis.
  - Signal in the RAVE trial suggesting there may be a slight advantage to rituximab in relapsing disease.
- **Notes:**
  - In the RITUXVAS trial, both control and treatment groups were receiving cyclophosphamide.
  - Despite newer evidence, there is still disagreement on the preferred regimen.
  - Although some providers treat with both cyclophosphamide and rituximab, it is much less common and not favored by most providers.

PRACTICE

Plasmapheresis is primarily considered for ANCA renal vasculitis patients who have severe or rapidly declining renal function (Cr > 4.0), with high likelihood of need for dialysis.

Evidence

- **Source:** MEPEX Trial. Jayne DRW, Gaskin G, Rasmussen N, et al.; European Vasculitis Study Group. Randomized trial of plasma exchange or high-dosage methylprednisolone as adjunctive therapy for severe renal vasculitis. *J Am Soc Nephrol.* 2007;18(7):2180–8.
- **Source:** PEXIVAS Trial. Walsh M, Merkel PA, Peh CA, et al.; PEXIVAS Investigators. The effects of plasma exchange and reduced-dose glucocorticoids during remission-induction for treatment of severe ANCA-associated vasculitis. *N Engl J Med.* 2020;382:622–31.
- **Takeaways:**
  - Plasma exchange demonstrated no improvement in mortality or reduction of progression to ESRD.
  - Lower glucocorticoid doses were as effective as higher doses but with lower rates of serious infection.

- **Notes:**
  - Plasma exchange may decrease rituximab levels. Consult with pharmacy to schedule the Rituximab doses accordingly.

PRACTICE

The current standard therapy for anti-glomerular basement membrane disease is plasmapheresis with immunosuppressive therapy, typically cyclophosphamide and prednisone.

Evidence

- **Source:** Levy JB, Turner AN, Rees AJ, Pusey CD. Long-term outcome of anti-glomerular basement membrane antibody disease treated with plasma exchange and immunosuppression. *Ann Intern Med.* 2001;134(11):1033–42.
- **Takeaways:**
  - Retrospective review that observed the best chance of renal recovery in patients who were treated with rapid immunosuppression therapy (plasmapheresis, prednisolone, and cyclophosphamide)
- **Notes:**
  - Prednisone is converted by the liver to prednisolone, its active form.

PRACTICE

Group A streptococcus (GAS) infection is treated with antibiotics to reduce the probability of developing poststreptococcal glomerulonephritis (PSGN) and, if PSGN is already present, to reduce severity.

Evidence

- **Source:** Johnston F, Carapetis J, Patel MS, et al. Evaluating the use of penicillin to control outbreaks of acute poststreptococcal glomerulonephritis. *Pediatr Infect Dis J.* 1999;18(4):327.
- **Takeaways:**
  - Treatment of GAS infection with penicillin reduced the development of PSGN.
- **Notes:**
  - Treating GAS infection is known to prevent development of rheumatic fever but has classically been taught to medical students as having no ability to reduce PSGN development.

PRACTICE

ACEIs or ARBs are standard therapy for reducing proteinuria and slowing the rate of immunoglobulin A (IgA) nephropathy progression.

Evidence

- **Source:** Park HC, Xu ZG, Choi S, et al. Effect of losartan and amlodipine on proteinuria and transforming growth factor-beta1 in patients with IgA nephropathy. *Neprhol Dial Transplant.* 2003;18(6):1115–21.
- **Source:** HKVIN Trial. Li PK, Leung CB, Chow KM, et al.; HKVIN Study Group. Hong Kong study using valsartan in IgA nephropathy (HKVIN): a double-blind, randomized, placebo-controlled study. *Am J Kidney Dis.* 2006;47(5):751–60.
- **Source:** STOP-IgAN Trial. Rauen T, Eitner F, Fitzner C, et al.; STOP-IgAN Investigators. Intensive supportive care plus immunosuppression in IgA nephropathy. *N Engl J Med.* 2015;373:2225–36.

- **Takeaways:**
  - Inhibition of RAAS led to significant decreases in proteinuria and disease progression.
- **Notes:**
  - Goal is to reduce proteinuria to less than 1 g/day.
  - Degree of proteinuria is correlated with prognosis.

PRACTICE

Plasmapheresis is the gold standard treatment for thrombotic thrombocytopenic purpura (TTP).

Evidence

- **Source:** Rock GA, Shumak KH, Buskard NA, et al. Comparison of plasma exchange with plasma infusion in the treatment of thrombotic thrombocytopenic purpura. Canadian Apheresis Study Group. *N Engl J Med.* 1991;325(6):393.
- **Takeaways:**
  - Plasma exchange was superior to plasma infusion in treatment of TTP.
- **Notes:**
  - Small study so difficult to pinpoint mortality benefits, but the survival rate of patients who receive plasmapheresis is significantly higher than the 90% mortality rate that existed prior to plasmapheresis availability.

Hematology

Anemia/Transfusion Therapy

PRACTICE

The standard hemoglobin threshold for transfusion is 7 g/dL unless the patient has cardiac disease for which the threshold is 8 g/dL.

Evidence

- **Source:** TRICC Trial. Hébert PC, Wells G, Blajchman MA, et al. A multicenter, randomized, controlled clinical trial of transfusion requirements in critical care. Transfusion Requirements in Critical Care Investigators, Canadian Critical Care Trials Group. *N Engl J Med.* 1999 Feb 11;340(6):409–417.
- **Takeaways:**
  - ICU patients without active bleeding were randomized to either a hemoglobin goal of greater than 7 g/dL versus 10 g/dL.
  - The restrictive transfusion strategy had a 4.7% absolute reduction in 30-day mortality.
- **Notes:**
  - The term "cardiac disease" has been interpreted loosely to range from active cardiac disease (e.g., ischemia) to any pre-existing cardiac disease such as heart failure.
  - Be especially careful when transfusing liver patients with varices as over-transfusing can plump up the varices and lead to increased risk of rupture.
  - Though the TRICC study was performed in ICU (critically ill) patients, its results are taken to apply to non-critically ill patients as well.

PRACTICE

Erythropoietin and darbepoetin are not used to target a "normal" hemoglobin level in patients with anemia of CKD.

Evidence

- **Source:** CHOIR Trial. Singh AK, Szczech L, Tang KL, et al.; CHOIR Investigators. Correction of anemia with epoetin alfa in chronic kidney disease. *N Engl J Med.* 2006 Nov 16;355(20):2085–2098.

- **Source:** TREAT Trial. Pfeffer MA, Burdmann EA, Chen CY, et al.; TREAT Investigators. A trial of darbepoetin alfa in type 2 diabetes and chronic kidney disease. *N Engl J Med.* 2009 Nov 19;361(21):2019–2032.
- **Takeaways:**
  - The CHOIR study demonstrated increased mortality in patients treated with the EPO-stimulating agents to a higher hemoglobin.
  - The TREAT study did not show increased mortality but did increase risk of thrombo-embolic stroke.
- **Notes:**
  - EPO agents do have a role in patients who struggle to maintain hemoglobin levels above the transfusion threshold.

PRACTICE

IV iron is given to patients with heart failure with reduced ejection fraction and concomitant iron deficiency.

Evidence

- **Source:** FAIR-HF Trial. Anker SD, Colet JC, Filippatos G, et al.; FAIR-HF Trial Investigators. Ferric carboxymaltose in patients with heart failure and iron deficiency. *N Engl J Med.* 2009 Dec 17;361(25):2436–2448.
- **Takeaways:**
  - IV iron replacement with ferric carboxymaltose led to significant improvements in subjective improvement in symptoms (20% absolute increase), the 6-minute walk distance (improvement by 35 m), as well as NHYA class (17% absolute improvement).
- **Notes:**
  - IV iron can be given if ferritin is less than 100 ng/mL or if ferritin is 100 to 300 ng/mL with less than 20% transferrin saturation.
  - Patients need not be anemic; they simply need to be iron deficient!
  - Interestingly, the only formulation of IV iron that has shown benefit is ferric carboxymaltose.

Leukemias

PRACTICE

ATRA is near-curative treatment for patients with the APML subtype of AML.

Evidence

- **Source:** Tallman MS, Andersen JW, Schiffer CA, et al. All-trans-retinoic acid in acute promyelocytic leukemia. *N Engl J Med.* 1997 Oct 9;337(15):1021–1028.
- **Takeaways:**
  - Three hundred and forty-six patients with APML were randomly assigned to all-trans-retinoic acid versus standard chemotherapy (cytarabine plus daunorubicin).
  - Significant increase in disease-free survival and overall survival with ATRA
- **Notes:**
  - ATRA encompasses several complex mechanisms that all lead to increased apoptosis of malignant cells.

PRACTICE

High daily dose of anthracycline combined with cytarabine improves the rate of complete remission in AML.

Evidence

- **Source:** Fernandez HF, Sun Z, Yao X, et al. Anthracycline dose intensification in acute myeloid leukemia. *N Engl J Med.* 2009 Sep 24;361(13):1249–1259.
- **Takeaways:**
  - Patients who received high-dose daunorubicin had a higher rate of complete remission (70.6% vs. 57.3%).
  - No difference in rates of serious side effects
  - Both treatment arms included therapy on top of cytarabine
- **Notes:**
  - Daunorubicin functions by inhibition of topoisomerase II, thus preventing the progression of DNA replication.
  - Daunorubicin may cause cardiomyopathy.

PRACTICE

Imatinib is used as first-line therapy in newly diagnosed Philadelphia chromosome-positive CML.

Evidence

- **Source:** IRIS Trial. O'Brien SG, Guilhot F, Larson RA, et al.; IRIS Investigators. Imatinib compared with interferon and low-dose cytarabine for newly diagnosed chronic-phase chronic myeloid leukemia. *N Engl J Med.* 2003 Mar 13;348(11): 994–1004.
- **Takeaways:**
  - Imatinib resulted in 17.6% absolute increase in progression-free survival at 18 months.
  - Number needed to treat very impressive: 6
- **Notes:**
  - The Philadelphia chromosome results from a t (9;22) translocation that produces the BCR-ABL protein, which leads to an increase in cell proliferation.

PRACTICE

Ibrutinib combined with rituximab is an effective regimen in patients with previously untreated CLL.

Evidence

- **Source:** Shanafelt TD, Wang XV, Kay NE, et al. Ibrutinib-rituximab or chemoimmunotherapy for chronic lymphocytic leukemia. *N Engl J Med.* 2019 Aug 1;381(5):432–443.
- **Takeaways:**
  - Patients who received ibrutinib-rituximab had significantly better progression-free survival (89.4% vs. 72.9).
- **Notes:**
  - Ibrutinib reduces chemotaxis by inhibiting cellular adhesion.

Lymphomas

PRACTICE

The IPS score is used as prognostic indicator for advanced-stage Hodgkin's lymphoma.

Evidence

- **Source:** Moccia AA, Donaldson J, Chhanabhai M, et al. International Prognostic Score in advanced-stage Hodgkin's lymphoma: altered utility in the modern era. *J Clin Oncol.* 2012 Sep 20;30(27):3383–3388.
- **Takeaways:**
  - First study validating the IPS score for advanced-stage Hodgkin's lymphoma in the setting of newer therapies (hence improved outcome)
  - Five-year freedom from progression was 78% and overall survival was 90%.
- **Notes:**
  - For patients treated prior to 1992, the 5-year freedom from progression and overall survival ranged from 42% to 84% and 56% to 89%, respectively.

PRACTICE

The FLIPI score is used as a prognostic measure in patients with follicular lymphoma.

Evidence

- **Source:** Solal-Céligny P, Roy P, Colombat P, et al. Follicular lymphoma international prognostic index. *Blood.* 2004 Sep 1;104(5):1258–1265.
- **Takeaways:**
  - Patients included in this study were diagnosed with follicular lymphoma from 1985 to 1992.
  - Five risk factors were determined: age, Ann Arbor stage, hemoglobin level, number of nodal areas, and serum LDH level.
  - Three risk groups (low risk, intermediate risk, and poor risk) were defined.
- **Notes:**
  - The FLIPI is currently used to improve treatment choices, and it seems to be more discriminant than other prognostic indexes used in lymphomas.

PRACTICE

In patients with diffuse large B-cell lymphoma, the revised international prognostic index (R-IPI) provides improved prognostic information.

Evidence

- **Source:** Sehn LH, Berry B, Chhanabhai M, et al. The revised International Prognostic Index (R-IPI) is a better predictor of outcome than the standard IPI for patients with diffuse large B-cell lymphoma treated with R-CHOP. *Blood.* 2007 Mar 1;109(5):1857–1861.
- **Takeaways:**
  - With the advent of R-CHOP, a significant improvement in survival led to unreliability of the IPI in patients with diffuse large B-cell lymphoma.
  - Three new distinct prognostic groups were proposed based on new data relevant to R-CHOP survivors: very good, good, and poor.

Neutropenia/Neutropenic Fever

PRACTICE

In cancer patients with neutropenia, levofloxacin may be used temporarily to prevent bacterial infections until neutropenia resolves.

Evidence

- **Source:** Bucaneve G, Micozzi A, Menichetti F, et al. Levofloxacin to prevent bacterial infection in patients with cancer and neutropenia. *N Engl J Med.* 2005 Sep 8;353(10):977–987.
- **Takeaways:**
  - No difference in overall mortality with or without levofloxacin
  - Fever was significantly reduced (20% absolute) in the levofloxacin group.
  - Levofloxacin demonstrated fewer microbiologically documented infections (17% less) and bacteremia (16% less).
- **Notes:**
  - Prophylactic levofloxacin is typically continued until neutropenia improves to over 1000 neutrophils per cubic millimeter.

PRACTICE

In febrile cancer patients with neutropenia, voriconazole may be a well-tolerated alternative to amphotericin B for empiric fungal coverage.

Evidence

- **Source:** Walsh TJ, Pappas P, Winston DJ, et al.; National Institute of Allergy and Infectious Diseases Mycoses Study Group. Voriconazole compared with liposomal amphotericin B for empirical antifungal therapy in patients with neutropenia and persistent fever. *N Engl J Med.* 2002 Jan 24;346(4):225–234.
- **Takeaways:**
  - Similar treatment success with voriconazole (26%) versus amphotericin B (30.6%)
  - The voriconazole group had fewer cases of severe infusion-related reactions and nephrotoxicity.
- **Notes:**
  - Voriconazole is metabolized by hepatic cytochrome P450, thus has many drug interactions. Always check!

Polycythemia Vera

PRACTICE

Low-dose aspirin may be a relatively benign way to effectively reduce strokes in patients with polycythemia vera.

Evidence

- **Source:** Landolfi R, Marchioli R, Kutti J, et al.; European Collaboration on Low-Dose Aspirin in Polycythemia Vera Investigators. Efficacy and safety of low-dose aspirin in polycythemia vera. *N Engl J Med.* 2004 Jan 8;350(2):114–124.

- **Takeaways:**
  - Patients with polycythemia vera were randomized to receive 100 mg aspirin versus placebo.
  - The aspirin arm had a significantly reduced combined risk of nonfatal myocardial infarction, nonfatal stroke, or death from cardiovascular causes.
  - Overall mortality and cardiovascular mortality were not significantly different between the two groups.
  - No significant difference in major bleeding
- **Notes:**
  - The major cause of primary polycythemia vera is a mutation in the JAK2 gene, though this disease is usually not inherited.

PRACTICE

In patients with polycythemia vera, the goal hematocrit is 45% or less.

Evidence

- **Source:** CYTO-PV Trial. Marchioli R, Finazzi G, Specchia G, et al.; CYTO-PV Collaborative Group. Cardiovascular events and intensity of treatment in polycythemia vera. *N Engl J Med.* 2013 Jan 3;368(1):22–33.
- **Takeaways:**
  - Three hundred and sixty-five patients were randomized to target a hematocrit of either less than 45% versus 45% to 50%
  - At 31 months, the intensive group had 3.3% (absolute) fewer cardiovascular or major thrombotic events.
  - Incidence of major bleeding was similar between the two groups.
- **Notes:**
  - Treatment options to reduce hematocrit include phlebotomy, aspirin, and hydroxyurea.

Sickle Cell Disease
PRACTICE

Hydroxyurea is used in patients with sickle cell to reduce the frequency of vaso-occlusive crises.

Evidence

- **Source:** Charache S, Terrin ML, Moore RD, et al. Effect of hydroxyurea on the frequency of painful crises in sickle cell anemia. Investigators of the Multicenter Study of Hydroxyurea in Sickle Cell Anemia. *N Engl J Med.* 1995 May 18;332(20): 1317–1322.
- **Takeaways:**
  - Hydroxyurea led to lower rates of vaso-occlusive crises (2.5 events vs. 4.5 events).
  - Median time to first crisis with hydroxyurea was 3 months versus 1.5 months.
  - Significantly less transfusions required with hydroxyurea (25% absolute reduction)
- **Notes:**
  - Hydroxyurea causes a shift in gene expression via inhibition of ribonucleotide reductase that results in the increased production of fetal hemoglobin and decreased adult hemoglobin. This shift in proportions reduces the frequency of sickling.

Thrombocytopenia

PRACTICE

High-dose dexamethasone is first-line therapy in patients diagnosed with primary immune thrombocytopenia.

Evidence

- **Source:** Mithoowani S, Gregory-Miller K, Goy J, et al. High-dose dexamethasone compared with prednisone for previously untreated primary immune thrombocytopenia: a systematic review and meta-analysis. *Lancet Hematol.* 2016 Oct;3(10):e489–e496.
- **Takeaways:**
  - This was a meta-analysis of nine randomized trials.
  - At 14 days, dexamethasone had greater platelet recovery.
  - At 6 months, there was no difference in overall platelet count response.
- **Notes:**
  - In approximately 60% of ITP cases, antibodies against platelets can be detected, usually against glycoprotein IIb-IIIa.

PRACTICE

The 4T's score is used to determine the likelihood of heparin-induced thrombocytopenia.

Evidence

- **Source:** Lo GK, Juhl D, Warkentin TE, et al. Evaluation of pretest clinical score (4 T's) for the diagnosis of heparin-induced thrombocytopenia in two clinical settings. *J Thromb Haemost.* 2006 Apr;4(4):759–765.
- **Takeaways:**
  - Based on the 4T's score, patients were classified into high, intermediate, and low probability groups for HIT.
  - Low scores correlated with low probability of testing positive for HIT antibodies (only 1 of 64 had positive antibodies in this group).
- **Notes:**
  - The 4 T's include: the degree of Thrombocytopenia, the Timing of platelet drop, presence of Thrombosis, and additional causes of Thrombocytopenia.

Tumor Lysis Syndrome

PRACTICE

Rasburicase is used for patients who are at high risk for tumor lysis syndrome.

Evidence

- **Source:** Cortes J, Moore JO, Maziarz RT, et al. Control of plasma uric acid in adults at risk for tumor lysis syndrome: efficacy and safety of rasburicase alone and rasburicase followed by allopurinol compared with allopurinol alone—results of a multicenter phase III study. *J Clin Oncol.* 2010 Sep 20;28(27):4207–4213.
- **Takeaways:**
  - Rasburicase decreased uric acid levels more quickly and to a greater magnitude than allopurinol alone.

- Rasburicase was well-tolerated both independently as well as in sequential combination with allopurinol.
- **Notes:**
  - Rasburicase functions by turning uric acid into allantoin, an inactive substance, thus reducing uric acid levels.

Venous Thromboembolism

PRACTICE

The Wells Score is used as a cost-effective means of identifying patients in whom D-dimer testing would be suitable for the purpose of ruling out pulmonary embolism.

Evidence

- **Source:** Wells PS, Anderson DR, Rodger M, et al. Excluding pulmonary embolism at the bedside without diagnostic imaging: management of patients with suspected pulmonary embolism presenting to the emergency department by using a simple clinical model and d-dimer. *N Engl J Med.* 2001 Jul 17;135(2):98–107.
- **Takeaways:**
  - Using a clinical model, patients were categorized as likely or unlikely to have a pulmonary embolism prior to obtaining a D-dimer.
  - Among patients who were low-risk and received D-dimers, only one patient (0.1%) ended up having an undiagnosed pulmonary embolism.
- **Notes:**
  - Patients with a Wells Score of 0 or 1 have a 1.3% chance of a pulmonary embolism in an ED population.

PRACTICE

Low-molecular-weight heparin (LMWH) is effective at preventing venous thromboembolism.

Evidence

- **Source:** Decousus H, Leizorovicz A, Parent F, et al. A clinical trial of vena caval filters in the prevention of pulmonary embolism in patients with proximal deep-vein thrombosis. Prévention du Risque d'Embolie Pulmonaire par Interruption Cave Study Group. *N Engl J Med.* 1998 Feb 12;338(7):409–415.
- **Takeaways:**
  - The original intent of the study was to examine the benefit of IVC filters. Yet, by accidental design, it confirmed the use of low-molecular-weight heparin as a viable pharmacologic means of VTE prophylaxis.
  - LMWH had 1.6% of patients develop a PE versus 4.2% in the unfractionated arm.

PRACTICE

In cancer patients, LMWH is effective in reducing recurrent venous thromboembolism.

Evidence

- **Source:** Lee AY, Levine MN, Baker RI, et al.; CLOT Investigators. Low-molecular-weight heparin versus a coumarin for the prevention of recurrent venous thromboembolism in patients with cancer. *N Engl J Med.* 2003 Jul 10;349(2):146–153.

- **Takeaways:**
  - In the Comparison of Low Molecular Weight Heparin Versus Oral Anticoagulant Therapy for Long Term Anticoagulation in Cancer Patients with Venous Thromboembolism (CLOT) trial, patients were randomly selected to receive dalteparin versus warfarin.
  - Eight percent of patients had a recurrent VTE in the dalteparin arm versus 15.8% of patients in the warfarin arm.
  - Additionally, 14% of patients had any bleeding on dalteparin versus 19% on warfarin.
- **Notes:**
  - A major criticism of this trial was that patients who had received warfarin had a supra-therapeutic only INR 24% of the time.

PRACTICE

Rivaroxaban is a first-line therapy used to treat deep vein thrombosis and pulmonary embolisms.

Evidence

- **Source:** EINSTEIN-DVT Trial. EINSTEIN-DVT Investigators. Oral rivaroxaban for symptomatic venous thromboembolism. *N Engl J Med.* 2010 Dec 23;363(26):2499–2510.
- **Source:** EINSTEIN-PE Trial. EINSTEIN–PE Investigators. Oral rivaroxaban for the treatment of symptomatic pulmonary embolism. *N Engl J Med.* 2012 Apr 5;366(14):1287–1297.
- **Takeaways:**
  - For treatment of DVT, Rivaroxaban had noninferior efficacy with respect to the primary outcome (2.1% vs. 3.0%). In the continued-treatment study, rivaroxaban had superior (1.3% vs. 7.1%).
  - For treatment of PE, at a mean follow-up of 7 months, rivaroxaban was noninferior to standard therapy in terms of the rate of recurrent symptomatic VTE (2.1% vs. 1.8%) and had a similar risk of clinically significant bleeding (10.3% vs. 11.4%).
- **Notes:**
  - Rivaroxaban needs to be taken with food in order to achieve higher bioavailability (>80%).

PRACTICE

Apixaban is a first-line therapy used to treat deep vein thrombosis and pulmonary embolism.

Evidence

- **Source:** AMPLIFY Trial. Agnelli G, Buller HR, Cohen A, et al.; AMPLIFY Investigators. Oral apixaban for the treatment of acute venous thromboembolism. *N Engl J Med.* 2013 Aug 29;369(9):799–808.
- **Takeaways:**
  - At 6 months, apixaban was noninferior to warfarin/LMWH for prevention of recurrent VTE or VTE death.
  - Apixaban was associated with significantly less major bleeding compared to warfarin/LMWH (0.6% vs. 1.8%).
- **Notes:**
  - Apixaban is now approved for patients with end-stage renal disease and those on hemodialysis.
  - Unlike for atrial fibrillation, low-dose apixaban is not evidence-based for DVT/PE.

PRACTICE

Aspirin is used as secondary prevention of VTE after completion of treatment and resolution.

Evidence

- **Source:** ASPIRE Trial. Brighton TA, Eikelboom JW, Mann K, et al.; ASPIRE Investigators. Low-dose aspirin for preventing recurrent venous thromboembolism. *N Engl J Med.* 2012 Nov 22;367(21):1979–1987.
- **Source:** WARFASA Trial. Becattini C, Agnelli G, Schenone A, et al.; WARFASA Investigators. Aspirin for preventing the recurrence of venous thromboembolism. *N Engl J Med.* 2012 May 24;366(21):1959–1967.
- **Takeaways:**
  - Though nonsignificant, the aspirin arm in ASPIRE did show a close trend towards fewer VTE and cardiovascular events (4.8% vs. 6.5%; 5.2% vs. 8.0%, respectively).
  - WARFASA also demonstrated that aspirin was associated with fewer VTE recurrences (6.6% vs. 11.2% per year).
- **Notes:**
  - These two trials combined make a strong case for aspirin as secondary prevention in cases where patients have no significant contraindication to aspirin therapy (now a Grade IIb recommendation per the AHA).
  - Unlike ASPIRE, WARFASA patients had completed a minimum of 6 and maximum of 18 months of anticoagulation prior to starting the aspirin.

PRACTICE

Edoxaban is effective in the treatment of cancer-associated venous thromboembolism.

Evidence

- **Source:** Hokusai VTE Trial. Raskob GE, van Es N, Verhamme P, et al.; Hokusai VTE Cancer Investigators. Edoxaban for the treatment of cancer-associated venous thromboembolism. *N Engl J Med.* 2018 Feb 15;378(7):615–624.
- **Takeaways:**
  - Edoxaban was noninferior to the LWMH arm (7.9% vs. 11.3%).
  - Rate of major bleeding was higher in the edoxaban group (6.9% vs. 4.0%).
- **Notes:**
  - Edoxaban is the first DOAC to be used for cancer patients with venous thromboembolisms.

PRACTICE

Insertion of inferior vena caval filters is not routinely used as prophylaxis against pulmonary embolism.

Evidence

- **Source:** Decousus H, Leizorovicz A, Parent F, et al. A clinical trial of vena caval filters in the prevention of pulmonary embolism in patients with proximal deep-vein thrombosis. Prévention du Risque d'Embolie Pulmonaire par Interruption Cave Study Group. *N Engl J Med.* 1998 Feb 12;338(7):409–415.
- **Takeaways:**
  - The IVC filter group had 1.1% of patients develop a pulmonary embolism versus 4.8% in the anticoagulation-only group.

- Notably, after 2 years, 20.8% of patients with the filter had a recurrent DVT as opposed to 11.6% in the anticoagulation group.
- No overall difference in mortality
- **Notes:**
    - IVC filters may be permanent or retrievable. While the evidence is not clear-cut, permanent IVC filters are thought to be associated with lower risk of complications such as filter migration.
    - IVC filters are thought to increase the risk of clot formation given the flow of blood is disrupted when passing over the filter, thus contributing directly to Virchow's triad.

Oncology

Colorectal

PRACTICE

Colonoscopy and colonoscopic removal of adenomatous polyps is the gold standard and preferred method of screening for colorectal cancer.

Evidence

- **Source:** Zauber AG, Winawer SJ, O'Brien MJ, et al. Colonoscopic polypectomy and long-term prevention of colorectal-cancer deaths. *N Engl J Med.* 2012;366:687–696.
- **Takeaways:**
  - Fifty-three percent reduction in mortality when colonoscopy included polypectomy
- **Notes:**
  - Patients should be screened at least every 10 years in the absence of abnormal findings.

PRACTICE

Colonoscopy is routine practice in some countries for colorectal cancer screening, but its prevalence and effectiveness are unclear in other countries.

Evidence

- **Source:** Bretthauer M, Kaminski MF, Løberg M, et al. Population-based colonoscopy screening for colorectal cancer. *JAMA Intern Med.* 2016;176(7):894–902.
- **Takeaways:**
  - Good adenoma detection rates in both the proximal and distal colon
- **Notes:**
  - Common non-anesthesia-related side effects of colonoscopy include abdominal pain due to air insufflation.
  - This air insufflation can be reduced with carbon dioxide rather than oxygen.

PRACTICE

Annual or biannual fecal immunochemical testing (FIT) is an alternative colorectal cancer screening method in the setting of patient preference or a contraindication to colonoscopy.

Evidence

- **Source:** COLONPREV Trial. Quintero E, Castells A, Bujanda L, et al. Colonoscopy versus fecal immunochemical testing in colorectal-cancer screening. *N Engl J Med.* 2012;366(8):697–706.
- **Takeaways:**
  - FIT was noninferior to colonoscopy for colorectal cancer screening.
- **Notes:**
  - The 10-year follow-up on mortality will end this year (2021).

PRACTICE

Fecal occult blood testing (FOBT), though not the gold standard, may be performed for colorectal cancer screening in patients in lieu of colonoscopy.

Evidence

- **Source:** Allison JE, et al. A comparison of fecal occult-blood tests for colorectal-cancer screening. *N Engl J Med.* 1996;334:155–160.
- **Takeaways:**
  - This study focused on newer generation fecal occult-blood (guaiac) tests, namely the Hemoccult II Sensa and HemeSelect.
  - Sensitivity is generally low with FOBT, and the maximum sensitivity was with the Hemoccult II Sensa (79.4%).
  - Hemoccult II was the most specific test at 97.7%.
- **Notes:**
  - The yield of FOBT is likely significantly dependent on the operator. Thus, ensure that you are proficient in FOBT technique!

Breast

PRACTICE

Mammograms are part of routine screening for breast cancer starting at age 45 (American Cancer Society) or 50 (U.S. Preventive Services Task Force).

Evidence

- **Source:** UK Age Trial. Moss SM, Cuckle H, Evans A, et al. Effect of mammographic screening from age 40 years on breast cancer mortality at 10 years' follow-up: a randomised controlled trial. *Lancet.* 2006;368(9552):2053–2060.
- **Takeaways:**
  - No difference in mortality due to breast cancer between patients screened starting at age 40 versus 50
- **Notes:**
  - Originally, USPSTF guidelines recommended screening at age 40 but that was based on a questionable meta-analysis. The recommendation was downgraded in 2009, with a recommendation to individualize the initiation of screening in patients younger than 50.

PRACTICE

Axillary lymph node dissection is preferred when possible compared to sentinel lymph node biopsy due to the lower complication rate.

Evidence

- **Source:** NSABP B-32 Trial. Krag DN, Anderson SJ, Julian TB, et al. Sentinel-lymph-node resection compared with conventional axillary-lymph-node dissection in clinically node-negative patients with breast cancer: overall survival findings from the NSABP B-32 randomised phase 3 trial. *Lancet Oncol.* 2010 Oct;11(10):927–933.
- **Takeaways:**
  - No difference in mortality between axillary and sentinel lymph node resection
  - Sentinel lymph node biopsy associated with fewer procedural complications
- **Notes:**
  - Lymphedema is a relatively common complication of both, but more frequently sentinel lymph node, resections. It is characterized by asymmetric pitting edema of the entire upper extremity and may be mistaken for a DVT by clinicians unfamiliar with the patient's surgical history.

PRACTICE

Trastuzumab is first-line therapy in HER2-positive breast cancer therapy after adjuvant chemotherapy.

Evidence

- **Source:** HERA Trial. Piccart-Gebhart MJ et al. Trastuzumab after adjuvant chemotherapy in HER2-positive breast cancer. *N Engl J Med.* 2005;353(16):1659–1672.
- **Takeaways:**
  - Trastuzumab after adjuvant chemotherapy resulted in a 6.5% absolute reduction in 1-year disease-free survival.
  - Interestingly, in a 2-year follow-up, trastuzumab did not demonstrate a significant benefit in disease-free survival.
- **Notes:**
  - Trastuzumab works by inhibiting the function of the HER2 receptor. It also attracts host white cells to cells that overexpress HER2.

PRACTICE

Tamoxifen or raloxifene may be used in select high-risk patients to reduce the incidence of breast cancer.

Evidence

- **Source:** STAR Trial. Vogel VG et al. Effects of tamoxifen vs raloxifene on the risk of developing invasive breast cancer and other disease outcomes. *JAMA.* 2006;295(23):2727–2741.
- **Takeaways:**
  - No significant difference between tamoxifen and raloxifene in breast cancer prevention
  - Tamoxifen resulted in a significant increase in thromboembolic events.
- **Notes:**
  - Tamoxifen should not be given to patients who have an increased risk for thromboembolic events such as stroke, DVT, or PE.

Lung

PRACTICE

Lung cancer screening is recommended in patients ages 55 to 80 with at least a 30 pack-year smoking history and either current smoking or smoking within the past 15 years.

Evidence

- **Source:** NLST Trial. NLST Team. Reduced lung-cancer mortality with low-dose computed tomographic screening. *N Engl J Med.* 2011;365:395–409.
- **Takeaways:**
  - Compared to screening chest x-ray, low-dose CT significantly reduced (~20%) lung cancer mortality in patients at increased risk (as defined above).
- **Notes:**
  - Low-dose CT screening should be done annually in qualifying patients.

Infectious Diseases

Clostridium difficile Colitis

PRACTICE

Two-tiered *C. diff* testing is a relatively new protocol now favored by many hospitals.

Evidence

- **Source:** Sharp SE, Ruden LO, Pohl JC, et al. Evaluation of the C. Diff Quik Chek Complete Assay, a new glutamate dehydrogenase and A/B toxin combination lateral flow assay for use in rapid, simple diagnosis of clostridium difficile disease. *J Clin Microbiol.* 2010;48(6):2082–6.
- **Takeaways:**
  - Two-tiered *C. diff* testing has increased sensitivity and speed compared to traditional polymerase chain reaction (PCR) and toxigenic culture diagnosis.
- **Notes:**
  - Two-tiered testing tests for glutamate dehydrogenase and toxins A/B.
    - Both glutamate dehydrogenase and toxins A/B present = positive
    - Both glutamate dehydrogenase and toxins A/B absent = negative
    - Discordant results = proceed to second-tier testing (reflex PCR on toxin gene)
  - False negative test possible if stool is left for greater than 2 hours at room temp or frozen
  - Sample must be liquid/loose stool to run test.

PRACTICE

Oral vancomycin is used as first-line therapy for *C. diff* treatment.

Evidence

- **Source:** Johnson S, Louie TJ, Gerding DN, et al. Vancomycin, metronidazole, or tolevamer for *Clostridium difficile* infection: results from two multinational, randomized, controlled trials. *Clin Infect Dis.* 2014;59(3):345–54.
- **Takeaways:**
  - Oral vancomycin is superior (81.1% vs. 44.2%) to metronidazole for resolution of diarrhea and absence of severe abdominal discomfort for at least 2 consecutive days.
    - Severe *C. diff* infection resolution (78.5% vancomycin vs. 66.3% metronidazole)
- **Notes:**
  - Metronidazole is now a second-line agent added to PO vancomycin for treatment of severe *C. diff* infection.

PRACTICE

Fidaxomicin is used as an alternative to vancomycin for treatment of *C. diff*, primarily in the setting of recurrent *C. diff*. Use, however, is limited by cost.

Evidence

- **Source:** Louie TJ, Miller MA, Mullane KM, et al. Fidaxomicin versus vancomycin for *Clostridium difficile* infection. *N Engl J Med.* 2011;364(5):422–31.
- **Takeaways:**
  - Fidaxomicin is non-inferior to vancomycin for treating *C. diff* infection.
  - Fidaxomicin had a ~10% lower rate of recurrent *C. diff*.
- **Notes:**
  - Although the Infectious Diseases Society of America guidelines recommend either vancomycin or fidaxomicin as first-line agents for treatment of *C. diff*, vancomycin is favored given easier access and cheaper cost.

PRACTICE

Fecal microbiota transplant (FMT) is used as a therapeutic option for recurrent *C. diff* infection.

Evidence

- **Source:** van Nood E, Vrieze A, Nieuwdorp M, et al. Duodenal infusion of donor feces for recurrent *Clostridium difficile*. *N Engl J Med.* 2013;368(5):407–15.
- **Takeaways:**
  - Fecal transplant results in lower rates (81% vs. 31%) of recurrent *C. diff* infection compared to vancomycin.
- **Notes:**
  - Patient must typically have at least two recurrent *C. diff* infections before consideration for fecal transplant.

PRACTICE

Probiotics are not recommended as ancillary treatment of *C. diff* infection.

Evidence

- **Source:** PLACIDE Trial. Allen SJ, Wareham K, Wang D, et al. Lactobacilli and bifidobacteria in the prevention of antibiotic-associated diarrhea and *Clostridium difficile* diarrhea in older inpatients (PLACIDE): a randomised, double-blind, placebo-controlled, multicentre trial. *Lancet.* 2013;382(9900):1249–57.

- **Takeaways:**
  - Probiotics (specifically Lactobacillus acidophilus, Bifidobacterium bifidum, and Bifidobacterium lactis) do not reduce antibiotic or *C. diff*-associated diarrhea.
- **Notes:**
  - Probiotic therapy should be especially avoided in immunocompromised patients as there is a risk of fungemia.

Bacteremia

PRACTICE

Two to three blood cultures are typically obtained for workup of bacteremia.

Evidence

- **Source:** Washington JA. Blood cultures: principles and techniques. *Mayo Clin Proc.* 1975;50(2):91–8.
- **Takeaways:**
  - Bloodstream infection detection rates were 80%, 88%, and 99% for use of one, two, and three blood cultures, respectively.
- **Source:** Cockerill FR, Wilson JW, Vetter EA, et al. Optimal testing parameters for blood cultures. *Clin Infect Dis.* 2004;38(12):1724–30.
- **Takeaways:**
  - 95.7% of bloodstream infections were detected with the first three blood cultures.
- **Source:** Lee A, Mirrett S, Reller LB, Weinstein MP. Detection of bloodstream infections in adults: how many blood cultures are needed? *J Clin Microbiol.* 2007;45(11):3546–8.
- **Takeaways:**
  - Two independent blood cultures detected 90% of bloodstream infections.
- **Notes:**
  - Blood cultures should be drawn from independent locations.
  - All indwelling ports/lines (such as chemo ports) should have a blood culture drawn. If only one port/line grows positive cultures, this could indicate a port/line infection.
  - *Staphylococcus aureus* requires only one positive blood culture to be diagnostic for bacteremia.

PRACTICE

Beta-lactams (nafcillin, oxacillin, cefazolin) are used preferentially for the treatment of methicillin-susceptible *Staphylococcus aureus* (MSSA) bloodstream infections.

Evidence

- **Source:** McDaniel JS, Perencevich EN, Diekema DJ, et al. Comparative effectiveness of beta-lactams versus vancomycin for treatment of methicillin-susceptible *Staphylococcus aureus* bloodstream infections among 122 hospitals. *Clin Infect Dis.* 2015;61(3):361–7.
- **Takeaways:**
  - Beta-lactams are superior (35% lower mortality) to vancomycin for definitive treatment of MSSA bloodstream infections.
  - No difference in mortality with empiric treatment regimens
- **Notes:**
  - Vancomycin has a large molecular weight and does not penetrate the MSSA cell wall as effectively as beta-lactams, which are very small molecules.

PRACTICE

Rifampin is not used as adjunctive therapy for uncomplicated *S. aureus* bacteremia.

Evidence

- **Source:** ARREST Trial. Thwaites GE, et al. Adjunctive rifampicin for *Staphylococcus aureus* bacteremia (ARREST): a multicenter, randomised, double-blind, placebo-controlled trial. *Lancet.* 2018;391(10121):668–78.
- **Takeaways:**
  - No difference in mortality, treatment failure, or disease recurrence with the addition of rifampin in *S. aureus* bacteremia.
- **Notes:**
  - You can think of the primary indication for rifampin as adjunctive therapy in cases where there is increased risk for biofilm formation (e.g., in the presence of prostheses).

Infective Endocarditis

PRACTICE

The Modified Duke Criteria is used to diagnose infective endocarditis.

Evidence

- **Source:** Bayer AS, Ward JI, Ginzton LE, Shapiro SM. Evaluation of new clinical criteria for the diagnosis of infective endocarditis. *Am J Med.* 1994;96(3):211–9.
- **Source:** Li JS, Sexton DJ, Mick N, et al. Proposed modifications to the Duke criteria for the diagnosis of infective endocarditis. *Clin Infect Dis.* 2000;30(4):633–8.
- **Takeaways:**
  - The Modified Duke Criteria correlates well with clinical assessment by infectious disease experts.
- **Notes:**
  - In the case of *S. aureus* infection, only one positive blood culture is required.
  - The Modified Duke Criteria are designed for diagnosis of infective, not culture-negative or marantic, endocarditis.

PRACTICE

Infective native-valve endocarditis is empirically treated with vancomycin and ceftriaxone. Infective prosthetic-valve endocarditis is empirically treated with vancomycin, ceftriaxone, and gentamicin. This is to empirically cover most common causative organisms: *S. aureus*, Strep species, enterococcus as well as HACEK.

Evidence

- **Source:** Baddour LM, Wilson WR, Bayer AS, et al. Infective endocarditis in adults: diagnosis, antimicrobial therapy, and management of complications: a scientific statement for healthcare professionals from the American Heart Association. *Circulation.* 2015;132(15):1435–86..
- **Source:** Habib G, Hoen B, Tornos P, et al. Guidelines on the prevention, diagnosis, and treatment of infective endocarditis (new version 2009): the Task Force on the Prevention, Diagnosis, and Treatment of Infective Endocarditis of the European Society of Cardiology (ESC). Endorsed by the European Society of Clinical Microbiology and Infectious Diseases (ESCMID) and the International Society of Chemotherapy (ISC) for Infection and Cancer. *Eur Heart J.* 2009;30(19):2369–413.

- **Takeaways:**
  - There are no clinical trials or great studies that compare empiric antibiotic regimens for infective endocarditis. Practice is based on the consensus opinions of experts.
- **Notes:**
  - Always calculate glomerular filtration rate and assess renal function prior to initiating gentamicin.

PRACTICE

Rifampin is used as adjunctive therapy in the treatment of staphylococcal prosthetic valve endocarditis.

Evidence

- **Source:** Drinković D, Morris AJ, Pottumarthy S, et al. Bacteriological outcome of combination versus single-agent treatment for staphylococcal endocarditis. *J Antimicrob Chemother.* 2003;52(5):820–5.
- **Takeaways:**
  - Combination antibiotic therapy is 5.9× more likely to result in negative cultures for staphylococcal prosthetic valve endocarditis.
  - Combination antibiotic therapy was not superior to monotherapy for resulting in negative cultures in staphylococcal native valve endocarditis.
- **Notes:**
  - Rifampin is unique in that it has significant penetration into biofilm secreted by *S. aureus.*

Osteomyelitis

PRACTICE

Foot ulcers, particularly diabetic, that probe to bone or fail to heal, warrant evaluation for osteomyelitis.

Evidence

- **Source:** Newman LG, Waller J, Palestro CJ, et al. Unsuspected osteomyelitis in diabetic foot ulcers. Diagnosis and monitoring by leukocyte scanning with indium in 111 oxyquinoline. *JAMA.* 1991;266(9):1246–51.
- **Takeaways:**
  - All (diabetic) foot ulcers exposed to bone were complicated by osteomyelitis, suggesting a need for increased suspicion for osteomyelitis when bone is exposed.
  - The majority of these osteomyelitis cases were clinically silent without signs of infection or inflammation.
- **Notes:**
  - Diagnostic options include bone biopsy (gold standard), plain films, MRI, and leukocyte scanning (lower risk).

PRACTICE

In the absence of an alternate explanation, probing to bone in an ulcer is diagnostic for osteomyelitis.

Evidence

- **Source:** Grayson ML, Gibbons GW, Balogh K, et al. Probing to bone in infected pedal ulcers. A clinical sign of underlying osteomyelitis in diabetic patients. *JAMA.* 1995;273(9):721–3.

- **Takeaways:**
  - Further testing is unnecessary for the diagnosis of osteomyelitis if an ulcer probes to bone (specificity 85%, positive predictive value 89%).
- **Notes:**
  - Diagnostics including culture and bone pathology to determine the causative organism, sensitivities, and bone margins is still warranted.

PRACTICE

Workup of osteomyelitis involves a probe to bone test, ESR, plain X-rays, MRI, and examination of the ulcer size.

Evidence

- **Source:** Butalia S, Palda VA, Sargeantet RJ, et al. Does this patient with diabetes have osteomyelitis of the lower extremity? *JAMA.* 2008;299(7):806–13.
- **Takeaways:**
  - Meta-analysis revealed the best predictive factors for osteomyelitis in diabetics as ulcer area greater than 2 cm², probing to bone, ESR greater than 70, and abnormal plain film.
  - Negative MRI had a LR 0.14 for osteomyelitis.
- **Notes:**
  - Probe to bone is considered diagnostic for osteomyelitis.
  - Erythrocyte sedimentation rate/C-reactive protein are markers often obtained during treatment to support resolution.
  - Plain films do not demonstrate changes early on thus indicating that the lesion is greater than 2 weeks old. MRI picks up earlier evolving lesions.

PRACTICE

Osteomyelitis is initially treated with IV antibiotics followed by either oral or IV therapy.

Evidence

- **Source:** Li HK, Rombach I, Zambellas R, et al.; OVIVA Trial. Oral versus intravenous antibiotics for bone and joint infection. *N Engl J Med.* 2019;380(5):425–36.
- **Takeaways:**
  - Oral antibiotic therapy for osteomyelitis was non-inferior for treatment failure at 1 year compared to intravenous antibiotics of similar duration (6 weeks) when used after initial IV therapy.
  - *S. aureus* bacteremia is a notable exclusion criteria.
- **Notes:**
  - Bioavailability and penetration of antibiotics to bone should always be considered!
  - Antimicrobials without good bone penetration (fewer to remember this way):
    - Penicillin, metronidazole
  - PO antimicrobials with good PO bioavailability:
    - Clindamycin, doxycycline, linezolid, fluoroquinolones, Bactrim
    - Metronidazole, fluconazole

PRACTICE

The optimal duration of antibiotic therapy for chronic osteomyelitis is 6 weeks.

Evidence

- **Source:** Goldstein E, Spellberg B, Lipsky BA, et al. Systemic antibiotic therapy for chronic osteomyelitis in adults. *Clin Infect Dis.* 2012;54(3): 93–407.
- **Takeaways:**
  - No definitive studies suggesting clear guidelines on optimal duration of antibiotic therapy for chronic osteomyelitis. However, there is currently no evidence to suggest that antibiotic therapy for greater than 4 to 6 weeks achieves better clinical outcomes.
- **Notes:**
  - Antibiotic duration should be determined in conjunction with an infectious diseases specialist but typical course is minimum of 6 weeks but often longer for vertebral osteomyelitis or methicillin-resistant *Staphylococcus aureus* (MRSA) infection.
  - Amputation of affected bone often requires a shorter course of antibiotics especially if bone pathology confirms negative margins.

PRACTICE

Fluoroquinolones are a common PO option for osteomyelitis.

Evidence

- **Source:** Karamanis EM, Matthaiou DK, Moraitis LI, Falagas ME. Fluoroquinolones versus beta-lactam based regimens for the treatment of osteomyelitis: a meta-analysis of randomized controlled trials. *Spine.* 2008;33(10):E297–304.
- **Takeaways:**
  - Fluoroquinolones are equivalent to beta-lactams for treatment of osteomyelitis based on rates of treatment success, relapses, and adverse effects.
- **Notes:**
  - Rather than providing several studies, this meta-analysis does the best job of summarizing the data across seven RCTs.

Urinary Tract Infection

PRACTICE

Asymptomatic patients should not be screened for catheter-associated urinary tract infections (UTIs).

Evidence

- **Source:** Tambyah PA, Maki DG. Catheter-associated urinary tract infection is rarely symptomatic: a prospective study of 1,497 catheterized patients. *Arch Intern Med.* 2000;160(5):678–82.
- **Takeaways:**
  - Though CAUTIs are a source of antibiotic-resistant organisms, they rarely lead to bloodstream infections.
- **Source:** Leone M, Perrin AS, Granier I, et al. A randomized trial of catheter change and short course of antibiotics for asymptomatic bacteriuria in catheterized ICU patients. *Intensive Care Med.* 2007;33(4):726–9.
- **Takeaways:**
  - Treatment of an asymptomatic CAUTI does not reduce rate of urosepsis.
- **Notes:**
  - All catheters should be removed as soon as possible.

PRACTICE

Older patients with febrile UTI and no other obvious infection should be considered for bacteremia.

Evidence

- **Source:** Lee H, Lee YS, Jeong R, et al. Predictive factors of bacteremia in patients with febrile urinary tract infection: an experience at a tertiary care center. *Infection.* 2014;42(4):669–74.
- **Takeaways:**
  - 32.6% of patients with febrile UTI were bacteremic.
- **Notes:**
  - *S. aureus* in the urine is atypical and should immediately prompt workup to exclude bacteremia.

Tuberculosis

PRACTICE

QuantiFERON-TB Gold testing is used in patients with Bacillus Calmette–Guérin (BCG) vaccination.

Evidence

- **Source:** Pai M, Zwerling A, Menzies D. Systematic review: T-cell–based assays for the diagnosis of latent tuberculosis infection: an update. *Ann Intern Med.* 2010;149(3):177–84.
- **Source:** Diel R, et al. Negative and positive predictive value of a whole-blood interferon-γ release assay for developing active tuberculosis: an update. *Am J Respir Crit Care Med.* 2011;183(1):88–95.
- **Takeaways:**
  - QuantiFERON-TB Gold testing had higher specificity than tuberculosis (TB)-skin testing for identification of latent TB in patients with BCG vaccination.
- **Notes:**
  - T-SPOT.TB testing is an alternative method that appears more sensitive than both TB skin and QuantiFERON testing.

PRACTICE

Adenosine deaminase (ADA) determination is used as a quick and reliable test for peritoneal TB.

Evidence

- **Source:** Riquelme A, Calvo M, Salech F, et al. Value of adenosine deaminase (ADA) in ascitic fluid for the diagnosis of tuberculous peritonitis: a meta-analysis. *J Clin Gastroenterol.* 2006;40(8):705–10.
- **Takeaways:**
  - ADA cutoff of 36 to 40 IU/L had 100% sensitivity and 97% specificity for peritoneal TB.
- **Notes:**
  - Cutoff ADA of 39 IU/L is recommended for clinical practice.

HIV/AIDS

Given the number of trials related to specific HIV antiretroviral therapies (ARTs), we instead cover the studies that guide our diagnosis and treatment principles. Knowledge about the evidence behind specific ART is beyond the detail that you will need to know unless specializing in HIV.

PRACTICE

Fourth generation combined antibody/antigen (HIV-1/2, P24) testing is the first-line diagnostic modality for HIV screening.

Evidence

- **Source:** Sickinger E, Jonas G, Yem AW, et al. Performance evaluation of the new fully automated human immunodeficiency virus antigen-antibody combination assay designed for blood screening. *Transfusion.* 2008;48(4):584–93.
- **Takeaways:**
  - Fourth generation antigen/antibody testing reduces the window period, allowing for earlier detection with 99.95% specificity.
- **Notes:**
  - All positive tests should be verified by the HIV1/2 differentiation assay.

PRACTICE

ART is initiated early regardless of CD4 count.

Evidence

- **Source:** NA-ACCORD Trial. Kitahata MM, Gange SJ, Abraham AG, et al. Effect of early vs. deferred antiretroviral therapy for HIV on survival. *N Engl J Med.* 2009; 360:1815–26.
- **Source:** INSIGHT START Trial. The INSIGHT START Study Group; Lundgren JD, Babiker AG, Gordin F, et al. Initiation of antiretroviral therapy in early asymptomatic HIV infection. *N Engl J Med.* 2015;373(9):795–807.
- **Takeaways:**
  - Early ART initiation defined as CD4+ greater than 500 decreased mortality and led to fewer complications.
- **Source:** Zolopa A, Andersen J, Powderly W, et al. Early antiretroviral therapy reduces AIDS progression/death in individuals with acute opportunistic infections: a multicenter randomized strategy trial. *PLoS One.* 2009;4(5):e5575.
- **Takeaways:**
  - Early ART in patients with AIDS-defining opportunistic infections led to decreased mortality and AIDS progression.
  - No increase in adverse effects or loss of virologic response
- **Notes:**
  - Transmission of HIV may also be reduced with early ART (HPTN 052 Trial).
  - All patients diagnosed with HIV should be offered ART with goal of viral suppression.

PRACTICE

Many providers now push for ART initiation on the same day as HIV diagnosis prior to availability of genotyping data.

Evidence

- **Source:** Pilcher CD, Ospina-Norvell C, Dasgupta A, et al. The effect of same-day observed initiation of antiretroviral therapy on HIV viral load and treatment outcomes in a US public health setting. *J Acquir Immune Defic Syndr.* 2017;74(1):44–51.

PRACTICE

Antibiotics should be initiated as soon as possible, preferably after obtaining diagnostics for future therapeutic guidance. If any delay in LP is anticipated, obtain blood cultures and initiate empiric antibiotics.

Evidence

- **Source:** Aronin SI, Peduzzi P, Quagliarello VJ. Community-acquired bacterial meningitis: risk stratification for adverse clinical outcome and effect of antibiotic timing. *Ann Intern Med.* 1998;129(11):862–9.
- **Source:** Proulx N, Fréchette D, Toye B, et al. Delays in the administration of antibiotics are associated with mortality from adult acute bacterial meningitis. *QJM.* 2005;98(4):291–8.
- **Takeaways:**
  - Delayed antibiotic therapy was associated with increased mortality.
- **Notes:**
  - Always consult with ID when there is high suspicion for meningitis!
  - Empiric antibiotics for age less than 50 ceftriaxone 2 g IV q12/vancomycin and dexamethasone to cover *S. pneumo*, meningococcus, *Haemophilus influenzae.*
  - Empiric antibiotics age greater than 50 ampicillin, ceftriaxone, and vancomycin to also cover listeria

PRACTICE

Dexamethasone should be initiated early for suspected bacterial meningitis.

Evidence

- **Source:** Gans J, van de Beek D; European Dexamethasone in Adulthood Bacterial Meningitis Study Investigators. Dexamethasone in adults with bacterial meningitis. *N Engl J Med.* 2002;347(20):1549–56.
- **Takeaways:**
  - Dexamethasone decreased mortality (relative risk [RR] 0.48) and unfavorable outcomes (RR 0.59) in bacterial meningitis.
  - No increase in GI bleeding risk.
- **Notes:**
  - The results of the study were driven by the *Streptococcus pneumoniae* patients and thus many believe that dexamethasone is most useful for pneumococcal meningitis.
  - Though dexamethasone did not demonstrate a benefit for hearing loss and neurologic sequelae in this study, other studies have suggested benefit.

Spontaneous Bacterial Peritonitis

PRACTICE

Patients with spontaneous bacterial peritonitis (SBP) are put on lifetime antibiotic prophylaxis.

Evidence

- **Source:** Rolachon A, Cordier L, Bacq Y, et al. Ciprofloxacin and long-term prevention of spontaneous bacterial peritonitis: results of a prospective controlled trial. *Hepatology.* 1995;22(4 Pt 1):1171–4.
- **Takeaways:**
  - Significant decrease in SBP (3.6% vs. 22%) for patients on ciprofloxacin prophylaxis.

- **Notes:**
    - Since this concept was first introduced, prophylaxis regimens have extended beyond fluo-roquinolones due to rising resistance rates. Despite that, ciprofloxacin 500 mg QD is among the most popular regimens.

PRACTICE

Nonselective beta-blockers (NSBBs) are discontinued in the setting of SBP.

Evidence

- **Source:** Mandorfer M, Bota S, Schwabl P, et al. Nonselective β blockers increase risk for hepatorenal syndrome and death in patients with cirrhosis and spontaneous bacterial peritonitis. *Gastroenterology.* 2014;146(7):1680-90.e1.
- **Takeaways:**
    - NSBBs increased the risk of acute kidney injury and hepatorenal syndrome.
- **Notes:**
    - Selective beta blockers may be continued with close monitoring.

Pneumonia

PRACTICE

CURB-65 scoring is commonly used to decide on inpatient versus outpatient treatment of community-acquired pneumonia (CAP).

Evidence

- **Source:** Lim WS, van der Eerden MM, Laing R, et al. Defining community acquired pneumonia severity on presentation to hospital: an international derivation and validation study. *Thorax.* 2003;58(5):377–82.
- **Takeaways:**
    - The CURB-65 scoring system was derived and validated in 1068 patients.
    - CURB-65 stratified patients into groups by mortality rates based on initial hospital assessment parameters.
- **Notes:**
    - The primary advantage of the CURB-65 over the Pneumonia Severity Index (PSI) is its ease of use. While PSI is slightly more accurate, it does rely on invasive testing such as an ABG.

PRACTICE

PSI is an alternative scoring system preferred by some physicians due to its more accurate prediction of mortality for CAP than CURB-65.

Evidence

- **Source:** Aujesky D, Auble TE, Yealy DM, et al. Prospective comparison of three validated prediction rules for prognosis in community-acquired pneumonia. *Am J Med.* 2005;118(4):384–92.
- **Takeaways:**
    - PSI had a better ability to discriminate short-term mortality and identify low-risk CAP patients than CURB-65.
- **Notes:**
    - Which system you use is often a matter of institutional preference.

PRACTICE

Antibiotics are initiated as soon as possible for cases of CAP.

Evidence

- **Source:** Daniel P, Rodrigo C, Mckeever TM, et al. Time to first antibiotic and mortality in adults hospitalised with community-acquired pneumonia: a matched-propensity analysis. *Thorax.* 2016;71(6):568–70.
- **Takeaways:**
  - Lower 30-day inpatient mortality (adjusted odds ratio 0.84) for CAP patients who received antibiotics within 4 hours of presentation
- **Notes:**
  - Without obvious contraindications, many clinicians opt to treat empirically since no pathogen is identified in the majority of cases
  - Unclear whether the mortality benefit is due to the antibiotic timing or rather reflects better care

PRACTICE

Empiric coverage for CAP includes atypical organism coverage.

Evidence

- **Source:** Arnold FW, Summersgill JT, Lajoie AS, et al. A worldwide perspective of atypical pathogens in community-acquired pneumonia. *Am J Resir Crit Care Med.* 2007;175(10):1086–93.
- **Takeaways:**
  - Atypical coverage resulted in 4% improved total mortality and decreased length of hospitalization by 1 day.
  - In North America, Europe, Latin America, Asia, and Africa, atypical organism incidence was approximately 20% to 28%.
- **Notes:**
  - Azithromycin predominantly covers for Strep and atypical organisms, thus coverage should be added for Staph infection if suspected.

PRACTICE

Severe CAP warrants consideration of combination antibiotic therapy with macrolides.

Evidence

- **Source:** Martinez JA, Horcajada JP, Almela M, et al. Addition of a macrolide to a beta-lactam-based empirical antibiotic regimen is associated with lower in-hospital mortality for patients with bacteremic pneumococcal pneumonia. *Clin Infect Dis.* 2003; 36(4):389–95.
- **Source:** Restrepo MI, Mortensen EM, Waterer GW, et al. Impact of macrolide therapy on mortality for patients with severe sepsis due to pneumonia. *Eur Respir J.* 2009; 33(1):153–9.
- **Takeaways:**
  - In severe CAP, macrolides have been associated with decreased mortality.
- **Notes:**
  - Severe CAP should never be treated with macrolide monotherapy!

PRACTICE

Given the increased side effects of fluoroquinolones, a shorter 5-day duration of 750 mg QD levofloxacin is preferred to a 10-day course of levofloxacin 500 mg QD.

Evidence

- **Source:** Dunbar LM, Wunderink RG, Habib MP, et al. High-dose, short-course levofloxacin for community-acquired pneumonia: a new treatment paradigm. *Clin Infect Dis.* 2003;37(6):752–60.
- **Takeaways:**
    - Levofloxacin 750 mg QD ×5 days was non-inferior to levofloxacin 500 mg QD ×10 days (92.4% vs. 91.1% clinical success rates).

PRACTICE

IV antibiotics for CAP treatment are converted to PO when patient is clinically improving and the patient is typically discharged with minimal observation after transitioning.

Evidence

- **Source**: Rhew DC, Hackner D, Henderson L, et al. The clinical benefit of in-hospital observation in "low-risk" pneumonia patients after conversion from parenteral to oral antimicrobial therapy. *Chest.* 1998;113(1):142–6.
- **Takeaways:**
    - Readmission rate for recurrent pneumonia was 5% in the non-observed group versus 2% in the observed group.
- **Notes:**
    - There is no clear benefit to observing the patient for a full 24 hours prior to d/c though many clinicians opt to observe for a short period.

Influenza

PRACTICE

Steroids are avoided in the setting of influenza due to increased mortality.

Evidence

- **Source:** Rodrigo C, Leonardi-Bee J, Nguyen-Van-Tam JS, Lim WS. Effect of corticosteroid therapy on influenza-related mortality: a systematic review and meta-analysis. *J Infect Dis.* 2014;212(2):183–94.
- **Takeaways:**
    - Review of 16 studies suggested an association of increased mortality with steroid administration in influenza infection.
- **Notes:**
    - No evidence from RCTs

PRACTICE

Oseltamivir is used to shorten the course of influenza in hospitalized or severely ill patients.

Evidence

- **Source:** Hernan MA, Lipsitch M. Oseltamivir and risk of lower respiratory tract complications in patients with flu symptoms: a meta-analysis of eleven randomized clinical trials. *Clin Infect Dis.* 2011;53(3):277–9.
- **Takeaways:**
  - 37% reduction in rate of lower respiratory tract complications requiring antibiotic treatment in patients confirmed for influenza infection
- **Notes:**
  - This was a review of 11 RCTs.
  - Oseltamivir is ideally given within 48 hours of symptom onset.

Procalcitonin

PRACTICE

Procalcitonin (PCT) is used at some institutions for clues to a bacterial lower respiratory tract infection.

Evidence

- **Source:** ProHOSP Trial. Schuetz P, Christ-Crain M, Thomann R, et al.; ProHOSP Study Group. Effect of procalcitonin-based guidelines vs standard guidelines on antibiotic use in lower respiratory tract infections: the ProHOSP randomized controlled trial. *JAMA.* 2009;302(10):1059–66.
- **Takeaways:**
  - PCT-guided therapy resulted in a 32% to 65% reduction in antibiotic exposure duration.
  - 8% to 27% reduction in antibiotic prescription rates with PCT-guidance
  - Similar rates of adverse outcomes in PCT versus control groups (15.4% vs. 18.9%)
- **Notes:**
  - Procalcitonin is not affected by liver failure or immunosuppression.
  - Most of the evidence for procalcitonin use has been in identifying a bacterial cause of infection and guiding antibiotic discontinuation in lower respiratory infections.

PRACTICE

Procalcitonin is sometimes used in sepsis to determine antibiotic initiation and cessation.

Evidence

- **Source:** PRORATA Trial. Bouadma L, Luyt CE, Tubach F, et al.; PRORATA trial group. Use of procalcitonin to reduce patients' exposure to antibiotics in intensive care units (PRORATA trial): a multicentre randomised controlled trial. *Lancet.* 2010;375(9713):463–74.
- **Takeaways:**
  - Antimicrobial use in severely ill ICU patients decreased with PCT-guided therapy without a significant increase in mortality.
- **Notes:**
  - There are no hard guidelines on exactly how to use procalcitonin and it is largely institution- and provider-dependent.

Skin and Soft Tissue Infections

PRACTICE

Non-purulent cellulitis does not require empiric MRSA coverage.

Evidence

- **Source:** Pallin DJ, Binder WD, Allen MB, et al. Clinical trial: comparative effectiveness of cephalexin plus trimethoprim-sulfamethoxazole versus cephalexin alone for treatment of uncomplicated cellulitis: a randomized controlled trial. *Clin Infect Dis.* 2013;56(12):1754–62.
- **Takeaways:**
  - No difference in treatment outcomes when treating non-purulent cellulitis with or without MRSA coverage.
- **Notes:**
  - The primary distinguishing feature for initial treatment of cellulitis is considering purulent versus non-purulent. Purulence typically signifies staph infection whereas non-purulent cellulitis is predominantly caused by strep species.

PRACTICE

Clindamycin is added to treatment regimens for necrotizing fasciitis.

Evidence

- **Source:** Andreoni F, Zürcher C, Tarnutzer A, et al. Clindamycin affects group A *Streptococcus* virulence factors and improves clinical outcome. *J Infect Dis.* 2016;215(2):269–77.
- **Takeaways:**
  - Clindamycin improved necrotizing fasciitis clinical outcomes even in clindamycin-resistant Group A strep.
- **Notes:**
  - Clindamycin inhibits production of key virulence factors by Group A strep.

Tick-borne Illnesses

PRACTICE

A single 200-mg dose of doxycycline is given prophylactically to patients with an Ixodes scapularis tick bite or engorgement.

Evidence

- **Source:** Nadelman RB, Nowakowski J, Fish D, et al. Prophylaxis with single-dose doxycycline for the prevention of Lyme disease after an *Ixodes scapularis* tick bite. *N Engl J Med.* 2001;345(2):79–84.
- **Takeaways:**
  - Single-dose doxycycline prophylaxis significantly reduced the rate of Lyme disease acquisition.
- **Notes:**
  - Woods and insect/tick exposure is a very easy, high-yield screening question for summer months in the Northeast.

PRACTICE

In the setting of suspected tick-borne disease, testing and empiric coverage should be provided for other tick-borne illnesses.

Evidence

- **Source:** Steere AC, McHugh G, Suarez C, et al. Prospective study of coinfection in patients with erythema migrans. *Clin Infect Dis.* 2003;36(8):1078–81.

- **Source:** Strickler RB, Gaito A, Harris NS, Burrascano JJ. Coinfection in patients with Lyme disease: how big a risk? *Clin Infect Dis.* 2003;37(9):1277–8.
- **Takeaways:**
  - Patients with Lyme disease were found to have between 4% and 28% co-infection rates with other tick-borne illnesses.
- **Notes:**
  - PO doxycycline to empirically cover for Lyme, anaplasmosis, and/or ehrlichiosis

PRACTICE

Due largely to ease of administration, PO doxycycline is the first-line treatment for early localized and disseminated Lyme disease (not including meningitis).

Evidence

- **Source:** Dattwyler RJ, Luft BJ, Kunkel MJ, et al. Ceftriaxone compared with doxycycline for the treatment of acute disseminated Lyme disease. *N Engl J Med.* 1997;337(5):289–94.
- **Takeaways:**
  - In early disseminated Lyme, PO doxycycline was equally as effective as IV ceftriaxone in preventing late-stage disease.
- **Notes:**
  - IV ceftriaxone is reserved primarily for Lyme meningitis and late disease.
  - Amoxicillin 500 mg TID is an alternative to PO doxycycline during pregnancy or if doxycycline is contraindicated (e.g., allergy).
  - Age less than 8 no longer a contraindication to doxycycline

PRACTICE

Transfusion and clindamycin are adjuncts used to treat severe babesiosis (typically defined as Hb <10, high-grade parasitemia [>10%], or evidence of end-organ damage).

Evidence

- **Source:** Hatcher JC, Greenberg PD, Antique J, Jimenez-Lucho VE. Severe babesiosis in Long Island: review of 34 cases and their complications. *Clin Infect Dis.* 2001; 32(8):1117–25.
- **Takeaways:**
  - Complicated babesiosis was more common when Hb less than 10 or parasitemia greater than 10%.
- **Notes:**
  - Clinical judgment should be utilized as there is limited data for precise transfusion requirements and each case has its own nuances.
  - RBC transfusion should reduce babesiosis parasitemia load by 50% to 90%.
  - Due to better tolerability many experts use atovaquone and azithromycin for severe babesia instead of clindamycin and quinine.

Invasive Fungal Infections

PRACTICE

Fluconazole prophylaxis is not routinely recommended for Cryptococcal infection.

Evidence

- **Source:** Sungkanuparph S, Savetamornkul C, Pattanapongpaiboon W. Primary prophylaxis for cryptococcosis with fluconazole in human immunodeficiency virus–infected patients with CD4 T-cell counts <100 cells/μL and receiving antiretroviral therapy. *Clin Infect Dis.* 2017;64(7):967–70.
- **Takeaways:**
  - After 2 years, there were no differences in either survival or new Cryptococcal infection rates.
- **Notes:**
  - No formal prophylaxis indicated for candidal infection either

PRACTICE

Voriconazole is first-line treatment for invasive aspergillosis.

Evidence

- **Source:** Herbrecht R, Denning DW, Patterson TF, et al. Voriconazole versus amphotericin B for primary therapy of invasive aspergillosis. *N Engl J Med.* 2002;347(6):408–15.
- **Takeaways:**
  - Voriconazole therapy of invasive aspergillosis had lower mortality and side effects than amphotericin B.
- **Notes:**
  - A common, important side effect of voriconazole is vision change.

Other Studies

PRACTICE

Universal MRSA decolonization protocols are now recommended in ICUs.

Evidence

- **Source:** REDUCE-MRSA Trial. Huang SS, Septimus E, Kleinman K, et al.; CDC Prevention Epicenters Program; AHRQ_DECIDE Network and Healthcare-Associated Infections Program. Targeted versus universal decolonization to prevent ICU infection. *N Engl J Med.* 2013;368(24):2255–65.
- **Takeaways:**
  - Universal decolonization of MRSA in ICUs is superior (37% reduction) to targeted decolonization.
  - MRSA bacteremia reduced by 28% (all-cause bacteremia by 44%)
- **Notes:**
  - MRSA decolonization is done via either nasal ointment (Bactroban/mupirocin) or chlorhexidine soap.

Endocrinology

Adrenal Gland Disorders

PRACTICE

A low morning cortisol can obviate the need for dynamic testing in patients with presumed adrenal insufficiency.

Evidence

- **Source:** Sbardella E, Isidori AM, Woods CP, et al. Baseline morning cortisol level as a predictor of pituitary-adrenal reserve: a comparison across three assays. *Clin Endocrinol (Oxf)*. 2017 Feb;86(2):177–184.
- **Takeaways:**
  - In this retrospective analysis, three of the most commonly used cortisol immunoassays were analyzed. This study found that the baseline cortisol levels for predicting with 100% specificity were 358 nmol/L for Siemens, 336 nmol/L for Abbott and 506 nmol/L for Roche.
- **Notes:**
  - These values convert to a range of 3.6 to 4.4 mcg/dL.

PRACTICE

Adrenal vein sampling is used to distinguish between unilateral adenoma and bilateral hyperplasia.

Evidence

- **Source:** Young WF, Stanson AW, Thompson GB, et al. Role for adrenal venous sampling in primary aldosteronism. *Surgery.* 2004;Dec;136(6):1227–1235.
- **Takeaways:**
  - In this study, patients with primary aldosteronism were selected based on degree of aldosterone excess, and CT findings. Both adrenal veins were catheterized in 194 patients (95.6%). Notable among the 110 patients with unilateral aldosterone hypersecretion were 41.4% patients with normal adrenal CT findings, 51.1% with unilateral micronodule (< or =10 mm) apparent on CT, 65.6% with unilateral macronodule (>10 mm) apparent on CT, 48.5% with bilateral micronodules, and 33% with bilateral macronodules.

- On the basis of CT findings alone, 42 patients (21.7%) would have been incorrectly excluded as candidates for adrenalectomy, and 48 (24.7%) might have had unnecessary or inappropriate adrenalectomy. AVS is an essential diagnostic step in most patients to distinguish between unilateral and bilateral adrenal aldosterone hypersecretion.
- **Notes:**
  - Continuous cosyntropin infusion is given during this procedure in order to minimize stress-induced fluctuations in aldosterone secretion as well as maximize the secretion of aldosterone from an adenoma.

PRACTICE

Adrenal incidentalomas greater than 4 cm should be considered for surgical resection.

Evidence

- **Source:** Mantero F, Terzolo M, Arnaldi G, et al. A survey on adrenal incidentaloma in Italy. Study Group on Adrenal Tumors of the Italian Society of Endocrinology. *J Clin Endocrinol Metab.* 2000 Feb;85(2):637–644.
- **Takeaways:**
  - This multicentric retrospective evaluation showed that mass size was the most reliable variable in separating benign from malignant adrenal incidentaloma. Masses greater than 4 cm had a 93% sensitivity in differentiating between benign and malignant tumors.
- **Notes:**
  - Imaging characteristics that suggest adrenal carcinoma or metastases include irregular shape, inhomogeneous density, high unenhanced CT attenuation values, and calcification.
  - In patients with unenhanced CT attenuation greater than 10 HU, pheochromocytoma should be excluded.

Diabetes Mellitus (Type I and Type II)
PRACTICE

Practitioners aim for a hemoglobin A1c goal of less than 7.0% in most patients with type II diabetes.

Evidence

- **Source:** Intensive blood-glucose control with sulfonylureas or insulin compared with conventional treatment and risk of complications in patients with type 2 diabetes (UKPDS 33). UK Prospective Diabetes Study (UKPDS) Group. *Lancet.* 1998 Sep 12;352(9131):837–853.
- **Source:** Gerstein HC, Miller ME, Byington RP, et al. Effects of intensive glucose lowering in type 2 diabetes. *N Engl J Med.* 2008 Jun 12;358(24):2545–2559.
- **Takeaways:**
  - In the 1998 UKPDS study, intensive glycemic control (fasting glucose <108 mg/dL) that reduces HbA1c by 11% over 10 years (median 7.0%) is associated with a 25% reduction in microvascular complications.
  - In the 2008 Action to Control Cardiovascular Risk in Diabetes (ACCORD) trial, intensive glycemic control (target HbA1c <6%) increases mortality compared to standard control (target A1c 7% to 7.9%).
- **Notes:**
  - There are numerous conflicting studies outlining the effects of intensive glucose control on macrovascular effects.

PRACTICE

Diabetic patients are treated with ace-inhibitors (Ace-I)/angiotensin II receptor blockers (ARBs) to help protect against diabetic nephropathy.

Evidence

- **Source:** Lewis EJ, Hunsicker LG, Bain RP, Rohde RD. The effect of angiotensin-converting-enzyme inhibition on diabetic nephropathy. The Collaborative Study Group. *N Engl J Med.* 1993 Nov 11;329(20):1456–1462.
- **Source:** Randomised placebo-controlled trial of lisinopril in normotensive patients with insulin-dependent diabetes and normoalbuminuria or microalbuminuria. The EUCLID Study Group. *Lancet.* 1997 Jun 21;349(9068):1787–1792.
- **Takeaways:**
  - In this randomized, controlled trial, diabetic patients with urinary protein excretion >/= 500 mg/day were either given captopril or placebo. The patients who had received captopril had a 50% reduction in the risk of combined end points of death, dialysis, and transplantation.
  - In a follow-up study in 1997, patients were either given lisinopril or placebo in patients with normoalbuminuria or microalbuminuria. Here, they showed that lisinopril slows the progression of renal disease in normotensive diabetes patients with little or no albuminuria, though the greatest effect was in those with microalbuminuria.
- **Notes:**
  - Similar effects have been seen in ARBs.

PRACTICE

In patients with pre-diabetes, lifestyle modification should be attempted prior to initiation of metformin in preventing the development of type II diabetes.

Evidence

- **Source:** Knowler WC, Barrett-Connor E, Fowler SE, et al. Reduction in the incidence of type 2 diabetes with lifestyle intervention or metformin. *N Engl J Med.* 2002 Feb 7;346(6):393–403.
- **Takeaways:**
  - In this randomized, controlled trial, pre-diabetic patients were assigned to either receive metformin or be enrolled in a lifestyle-modification program. Lifestyle changes and treatment with metformin both reduced the incidence of diabetes in persons at high risk. The lifestyle intervention was more effective than metformin.
  - The lifestyle intervention reduced the incidence by 58%, and metformin by 31%.
- **Notes:**
  - Per ADA Standard of Care Guidelines, pre-diabetics should be referred to a diabetic prevention program targeting a 7% weight loss and 150 minutes/week of moderate-intensity exercise.

PRACTICE

Diabetic patients are initiated on statin therapy based on their atherosclerotic cardiovascular disease (ASCVD) risk.

Evidence

- **Source:** Collins R, Armitage J, Parish S, et al. MRC/BHF Heart Protection Study of cholesterol-lowering with simvastatin in 5963 people with diabetes: a randomised placebo-controlled trial. *Lancet*. 2003 Jun 14;361(9374):2005.
- **Source:** Colhoun HM, Betteridge DJ, Durrington PN, et al. Primary prevention of cardiovascular disease with atorvastatin in type 2 diabetes in the Collaborative Atorvastatin Diabetes Study (CARDS): multicentre randomised placebo-controlled trial. *Lancet*. 2004;364(9435):685–696.
- **Takeaways:**
  - The Heart Protection Study (HPS) studied the effect of cholesterol lowering with simvastatin in specific patient groups with increased CVD risk. This includes patients with diabetes, CAD, peripheral artery disease (PAD), cerebrovascular disease, and hypertension. The trial randomized 20,536 patients to receive simvastatin 40 mg daily or placebo. The trial reported that cholesterol lowering was associated with reduced all-cause mortality (12.9% vs. 14.7% in placebo). In addition, a significant benefit on coronary mortality and other vascular mortality was evident. Simvastatin also reduced the risk of major vascular events (19.8% vs. 25.2%) in placebo.
  - The Collaborative AtoRvastatin Diabetes Study (CARDS) randomized 2383 diabetic patients to receive atorvastatin 10 mg daily or placebo. Atorvastatin reduced the risk of the primary outcome (ACS, coronary revascularization, or stroke) by 37% with a strong trend toward reduction of all-cause mortality risk (HR 0.73).
- **Notes:**
  - Per 2019 ACC/AHA guidelines, type II diabetic patients who are aged 40 to 75 should be initiated on a moderate intensity statin regardless of ASCVD score.

PRACTICE

While generally accepted for secondary prevention, aspirin is given to diabetic patients with an increased risk of ASCVD for primary prevention.

Evidence

- **Source:** Kunutsor SK, Seidu S, Khunti K. Aspirin for primary prevention of cardiovascular and all-cause mortality events in diabetes: updated meta-analysis of randomized controlled trials. *Diabet Med*. 2017 Mar;34(3):316–327.
- **Takeaways:**
  - A total of 10 randomized trials were included in this review. There was a significant reduction in risk of major adverse cardiovascular events: relative risk of 0.90 in groups taking aspirin compared with placebo or no treatment. However, limited subgroup analyses suggested that the effect of aspirin on major adverse cardiovascular events differed by baseline cardiovascular disease risk, medication compliance, and sex (P for interaction for all > .05). In addition, there was an increase in risk of major or gastrointestinal bleeding events, but estimates were imprecise and not significant.
- **Notes:**
  - Given the above data, aspirin should be considered in a diabetic patient with an ASCVD 10-year risk greater than 10%.

Obesity

PRACTICE

Naltrexone plus bupropion is effective in reducing weight in overweight and obese patients.

Evidence

- **Source:** Greenway FL, Fujioka K, Plodkowski RA, et al.; COR-I Study Group. Effect of naltrexone plus bupropion on weight loss in overweight and obese adults (COR-I): a multicentre, randomised, double-blind, placebo-controlled, phase 3 trial. *Lancet.* 2010 Aug 21;376(9741):595–605.
- **Takeaways:**
  - In this multicenter, randomized, placebo-controlled trial, patients who received naltrexone + bupropion had a mean change in body weight of 6.1 kg compared to matching placebo (1.4 kg) over a follow-up period of 56 weeks.
- **Notes:**
  - Relative contraindications are patients with uncontrolled hypertension, seizure disorder, chronic opioid use, bulimia, or anorexia nervosa.

PRACTICE

Bariatric surgery can lead to improvement in glycemic control in patients with type II diabetes.

Evidence

- **Source:** Chand B, Schauer PR. Can diabetes be surgically cured? Long-term metabolic effects of bariatric surgery in obese patients with type 2 diabetes mellitus. *Ann Surg.* 2013;Oct;258(4):628–636.
- **Takeaways:**
  - This study analyzed 217 type II diabetic patients who underwent bariatric surgery including sleeve gastrectomy, gastric banding, and roux-en-y gastric bypass between 2004 and 2007. Fifty percent of the patients achieved long-term complete (24%) or partial (26%) type II diabetes remission. Only 16% did not see improvement glycemic control, while the remaining 34% experienced improved glycemic control. Gastric bypass patients experienced more weight loss and lower diabetes remission rates than laparoscopic sleeve gastrectomy or laparoscopic gastric banding. Additionally, gastric bypass was associated with diabetes remission after multivariable analysis, along with shorter duration of diabetes and greater weight loss. Even patients with recurrence demonstrated improved diabetes metrics including significantly lower HbA1c, fasting blood sugar, and use of insulin. They also reached American Diabetes Association goals of glycemic control, blood pressure control, and LDL control in greater numbers.
- **Notes:**
  - Additionally, these patients had improved blood pressure and cholesterol control.

Osteoporosis

PRACTICE

In low-risk patients with stable bone mineral density, bisphosphonate therapy can be stopped after 5 years of therapy.

Evidence

- **Source:** Black DM, Schwartz AV, Ensrud KE, et al. Effects of continuing or stopping alendronate after 5 years of treatment: the Fracture Intervention Trial Long-term Extension (FLEX): a randomized trial. *JAMA.* 2006 Dec 27;296(24):2927–2938.
- **Takeaways:**
  - Compared with continuing alendronate, switching to placebo for 5 years resulted in declines in bone mineral disease at the total hip, but mean levels remained at

or above pretreatment levels. The cumulative risk of nonvertebral fractures was not significantly different between those continuing and those discontinuing alendronate.

- **Notes:**
  - Alendronate should be continued for up to 10 years in patients at highest risk for fracture (T-score below –3.5).

PRACTICE

In patients who are high risk for fractures who have difficulty with oral bisphosphonates or renal insufficiency, denosumab can be used as initial therapy.

Evidence

- **Source:** Cummings SR, San Martin J, McClung MR, et al. Denosumab for prevention of fractures in postmenopausal women with osteoporosis. *N Engl J Med.* 2009 Aug 20;361(8):756–765.
- **Takeaways:**
  - Denosumab given subcutaneously was associated with a reduction in the risk of vertebral, nonvertebral, and hip fractures in women with osteoporosis.
- **Notes:**
  - Denosumab inhibits receptor activator of nuclear factor kappa-B ligand, a protein involved with osteoclastogenesis.

Polycystic Ovarian Syndrome

PRACTICE

Metformin should not be used as first-line therapy in the treatment of polycystic ovarian syndrome.

Evidence

- **Source:** Costello M, Shrestha B, Eden J, et al. Insulin-sensitising drugs versus the combined oral contraceptive pill for hirsutism, acne and risk of diabetes, cardiovascular disease, and endometrial cancer in polycystic ovary syndrome. *Cochrane Database Syst Rev.* 2007 Jan 24;(1):CD005552.
- **Takeaways:**
  - In this meta-analysis, six trials were included for analysis, four of which compared metformin versus OCP (104 participants) and two of which compared OCP combined with metformin versus OCP alone (70 participants). Taken together, these data demonstrated no evidence of difference in effect between metformin and the OCP on hirsutism and acne. There was either insufficient or no data on the relative efficacy of metformin or the OCP (alone or in combination) for preventing the development of diabetes, cardiovascular disease, or endometrial cancer. Metformin was less effective than the OCP in improving menstrual pattern. Metformin was less effective in reducing serum androgen levels.
- **Notes:**
  - For women with oligomenorrhea who need endometrial protection, combined estrogen-progestin oral contraceptives should be used as first-line therapy. For management of hyperandrogenic symptoms alone, combined oral contraceptives are first-line therapy as well.

Parathyroid Diseases

PRACTICE

Patients with symptomatic primary hyperparathyroidism causing nephrolithiasis should undergo parathyroidectomy.

Evidence

- **Source:** Silverberg SJ, Shane E, Jacobs TP, et al. A 10-year prospective study of primary hyperparathyroidism with or without parathyroid surgery. *N Engl J Med.* 1999 Oct 21;341(17):1249–1255.
- **Takeaways:**
  - In this study, 61 patients underwent parathyroidectomy, and 60 patients were followed without surgery. Parathyroidectomy led to normalization of serum calcium. All the patients with a history of nephrolithiasis who did not choose to have parathyroidectomy had progression of disease.
- **Notes:**
  - Other clear indications for surgery include fractures and symptomatic hypercalcemia.

PRACTICE

Delayed technetium-99m sestamibi single photon emission computed tomography (SPECT) scans are used to facilitate a minimally invasive parathyroidectomy.

Evidence

- **Source:** Civelek AC, Ozalp E, Donovan P, Udelsman R. Prospective evaluation of delayed technetium-99m sestamibi SPECT scintigraphy for preoperative localization of primary hyperparathyroidism. *Surgery.* 2002 Feb;131(2):149–157.
- **Takeaways:**
  - SPECT imaging successfully detected 96% of solitary adenomas and 83% of double adenomas.
- **Notes:**
  - This imaging modality is limited in its evaluation of multiglandular hyperplasia (45% detected).

Thyroid Gland Disorders

PRACTICE

Medical, surgical, and radioiodine treatment for hyperthyroidism are equally effective in normalizing serum thyroid hormone concentrations.

Evidence

- **Source:** Törring O, Tallstedt L, Wallin G, et al. Graves' hyperthyroidism: treatment with antithyroid drugs, surgery, or radioiodine--a prospective, randomized study. Thyroid Study Group. *J Clin Endocrinol Metab.* 1996 Aug;81(8):2986–2993.
- **Takeaways:**
  - In this randomized prospective study, patients were assigned to receive anti-thyroid drugs for 18 months (medical), subtotal thyroidectomy (surgical), or radioiodine (iodine-131) treatment. Each was equally effective in normalizing serum thyroid hormone

concentrations within 6 weeks; after treatment, 95% of the patients were satisfied with their therapy.

- **Notes:**
  - Methimazole is the primary drug used (along with beta-blockers) to treat Graves' hyperthyroidism except during the first trimester of pregnancy (in which propylthiouracil is preferred).

PRACTICE

Third-generation TSH chemiluminometric is used to assess thyroid function.

Evidence

- **Source:** Ross DS, Ardisson LJ, Meskell MJ. Measurement of thyrotropin in clinical and subclinical hyperthyroidism using a new chemiluminescent assay. *J Clin Endocrinol Metab.* 1989 Sep;69(3):684–688.
- **Takeaways:**
  - Prior to this study, immunoradiometric assays were used. Using this third-generation chemiluminescent assay, sera were analyzed from 145 patients who had TSH concentrations below 0.08 mU/L in the immunoradiometric assay. Most patients with overt hyperthyroidism had undetectable TSH concentrations in the chemiluminescent assay. Three groups of patients were identified, in which a large subgroup had undetectable values in the immunoradiometric assay and detectable values in the chemiluminescent assay (12 of 17 patients under treatment for hyperthyroidism who had recently normalized their serum thyroid hormone levels, 33 of 68 patients taking L-T4, and 4 of 8 patients with endogenous subclinical hyperthyroidism).
- **Notes:**
  - This highly sensitive TSH test now allows us to distinguish degrees of thyrotrophic suppression in subclinical hyperthyroidism.

PRACTICE

Suspicious thyroid nodules are biopsied based on their ultrasound characteristics rather than size.

Evidence

Tang AL, Falciglia M, Yang H, et al. Validation of American Thyroid Association ultrasound risk assessment of thyroid nodules selected for ultrasound fine-needle aspiration. *Thyroid.* 2017 Aug;27(8):1077–1082.

- **Takeaways:**
  - The American Thyroid Association developed sonographic criteria for fine-needle aspiration (FNA) based on suspicious ultrasound features other than nodule size. These criteria correlated with the surgical pathology results.
- **Notes:**
  - Biopsy should be performed in nodules >= 1 cm with these suspicious features: irregular margins, microcalcifications, taller than wide shape, and rim calcifications.
  - FNA should be performed in nodules (regardless of size) with these features: extrathyroidal extension, subcapsular locations adjacent to the recurrent laryngeal nerve or trachea, extrusion through rim calcifications, or associated with cervical lymph nodes.

CHAPTER 11

Psychiatry

Core Psychiatry Tools

PRACTICE

The Montreal Cognitive Assessment (MOCA) is a commonly used screening tool for dementia.

Evidence

- **Source:** Nasreddine ZS, Phillips NA, Bédirian V, et al. The Montreal Cognitive Assessment, MoCA: a brief screening tool for mild cognitive impairment. *J Am Geriatr Soc.* 2005;53(4):695.
- **Takeaways:**
  - Scores less than 26 detected 90% of mild cognitive impairment subjects.
  - 100% specific for detecting mild Alzheimer's as opposed to 87%
- **Notes:**
  - Many studies have demonstrated that the MOCA test is more difficult than the MMSE.
  - Subsequent studies have suggested adding +1 to the overall score earned for formal education less than 12 years.

PRACTICE

The Mini-Mental Status Exam (MMSE) is a commonly used screening tool for dementia.

Evidence

- **Source:** Folstein MF, Folstein SE, McHugh PR. "Mini-mental state". A practical method for grading the cognitive state of patients for the clinician. *J Psychiatr Rev.* 1975;12(3):189.
- **Takeaways:**
  - Scores less than 20 were associated only with dementia.
- **Source:** Tsoi KK, Chan JYC, Hirai HW, et al. Cognitive tests to detect dementia: a systematic review and meta-analysis. *JAMA Intern Med.* 2015;175(9):1450.
- **Takeaways:**
  - Pooled sensitivity and specificity of 81% and 89%, respectively

- **Notes:**
  - 30-point scale with varying cutoffs, generally with scores less than 24 considered cognitively impaired
  - Originally developed for assessment of psychiatric patients

Major Depressive Disorder

PRACTICE

Cognitive behavioral therapy (CBT), a form of psychotherapy, is a first-line choice for major depressive disorder (MDD).

Evidence

- **Source:** Cuijpers P, Karyotaki E, Weitz E, et al. The effects of psychotherapies for major depression in adults on remission, recovery and improvement: a meta-analysis. *J Affect Disord.* 2014;159:118–26.
- **Takeaways:**
  - Remission of depression occurred in 41% of patients treated with CBT versus 21% in placebo.
  - No link between number of CBT sessions and overall impact on remission
- **Notes:**
  - CBT is a completely valid method of treatment although it may seem odd not to offer medications (namely, SSRIs)!
  - One challenge to CBT is finding therapists with expertise in CBT; however, there are an increasing number of providers who will do CBT remotely.

PRACTICE

For initial treatment of *mild* unipolar major depressive disorder (MDD), psychotherapy and pharmacologic therapy are equivocal.

Evidence

- **Source:** Cuijpers P, van Straten A, van Oppen P, Andersson G. Are psychological and pharmacologic interventions equally effective in the treatment of adult depressive disorders? A meta-analysis of comparative studies. *J Clin Psychiatry.* 2008;69(11):1675.
- **Takeaways:**
  - No significant difference in effectiveness of pharmacologic versus psychotherapy interventions for *mild* MDD
  - SSRIs (but not other antidepressant classes) significantly more effective in moderate to severe cases of MDD
- **Notes:**
  - Dysthymia is also known as persistent depressive disorder and *minor* depression.

PRACTICE

SSRIs are first-line pharmacologic treatment for major depressive disorder.

Evidence

- **Source:** Gibbons RD, Hur K, Brown CH, et al. Benefits from antidepressants: synthesis of 6-week patient-level outcomes from double-blind placebo-controlled randomized trials of fluoxetine and venlafaxine. *Arch Gen Psychiatry.* 2012;69(6):572.

■ **Source:** Arroll B, Elley CR, Fishman T, et al. Antidepressants versus placebo for depression in primary care. *Cochrane Database Syst Rev.* 2009;(3):CD007954.
■ **Takeaways:**
  ■ SSRIs are effective for treatment of MDD, with a median NNT of 7.
■ **Notes:**
  ■ Each trial of an SSRI and dosing should typically be several weeks.
  ■ Most SSRIs should be tapered gradually to prevent a flu-like withdrawal syndrome.

PRACTICE

SNRIs may be prescribed as first-line pharmacologic treatment for major depressive disorder.

Evidence

■ **Source:** Gibbons RD, Hur K, Brown CH, et al. Benefits from antidepressants: synthesis of 6-week patient-level outcomes from double-blind placebo-controlled randomized trials of fluoxetine and venlafaxine. *Arch Gen Psychiatry.* 2012;69(6):572.
■ **Source:** Girardi P, Pompili M, Innamorati M, et al. Duloxetine in acute major depression: review of comparisons to placebo and standard antidepressants using dissimilar methods. *Hum Psychopharmacol.* 2009;24(3):177–90.
■ **Takeaways:**
  ■ Duloxetine is effective in treating MDD at doses 80 to 120 mg QD.
■ **Notes:**
  ■ Lack of RCTs comparing duloxetine to other efficacious antidepressants
  ■ Duloxetine can also be used to treat neuropathic pain.

PRACTICE

Tricyclic antidepressants (TCAs) are second-line pharmacologic treatments for major depressive disorder.

Evidence

■ **Source:** Arroll B, Elley CR, Fishman T, et al. Antidepressants versus placebo for depression in primary care. *Cochrane Database Syst Rev.* 2009;(3):CD007954.
■ **Takeaways:**
  ■ TCAs are effective for treatment of MDD, with a median NNT of 9.
■ **Notes:**
  ■ TCAs may not be second line when other comorbidities (e.g., neuropathic pain) overlap with MDD.
  ■ Be careful of providing TCAs in patients with CAD.
  ■ Side effects (particularly anticholinergic effects such as dry mouth) can make titration of TCA doses challenging.

PRACTICE

Bupropion is a second-line treatment for major depressive disorder.

Evidence

■ **Source:** Reimherr FW, Cunningham LA, Batey SR, et al. A multicenter evaluation of the efficacy and safety of 150 and 300 mg/d sustained-release bupropion tablets versus placebo in depressed outpatients. *Clin Ther.* 1998;20(3):505–16.

- **Takeaways:**
  - Bupropion SR 150 mg was superior to placebo in improving depression rating scales in patients with MDD.
- **Notes:**
  - Lowers the seizure threshold
  - Some patients may experience "activation" by bupropion, thus this may not be the best choice for patients with depression and co-occurring anxiety.
  - Do not prescribe if patient has a history of eating disorders!
  - Less sexual dysfunction; good alternative for men experiencing erectile dysfunction

PRACTICE

Esketamine is a new class antidepressant recently approved by the FDA, but it is not currently recommended as first-line therapy.

Evidence

- **Source:** Daly EJ, Singh JB, Fedgchin M, et al. Efficacy and safety of intranasal esketamine adjunctive to oral antidepressant therapy in treatment-resistant depression: a randomized clinical trial. *JAMA.* 2018;75(2):139–48.
- **Takeaways:**
  - Intranasal esketamine had a rapid onset of action and was superior to placebo for improving depression rating scales (MADRS).
  - Antidepressant effect persisted for greater than 2 months.
- **Notes:**
  - Esketamine is the first antidepressant of the NMDA receptor antagonist class.
  - Esketamine's exact mechanism of action as an antidepressant is unknown.

PRACTICE

Sertraline is safe for use to treat MDD during acute coronary syndrome (ACS).

Evidence

- **Source:** SADHART Trial. Glassman AH, O'Connor CM, Califf RM, et al.; Sertraline Antidepressant Heart Attack Randomized Trial (SADHEART) Group. Sertraline treatment of major depression in patients with acute MI or unstable angina. *JAMA.* 2002;288(6):701–9.
- **Takeaways:** Sertraline is safe and effective for treatment of MDD in patients with recent acute coronary syndrome.
  - No significant effect on QT
- **Notes:**
  - Per a subgroup analysis, depression ratings improved among patients treated with sertraline who had MDD onset prior to recent ACS.

PRACTICE

Light therapy is reasonable first-line therapy for patients with seasonal affective disorder.

Evidence

- **Source:** Can-SAD Trial. Lam RW, Levitt AJ, Levitan RD, et al. The Can-SAD study: A randomized controlled trial of the effectiveness of light therapy and fluoxetine in patients with winter seasonal affective disorder. *Am J Psychiatry.* 2006;165(5):805–12.

- **Takeaways:**
  - Light therapy was associated with depression rating improvements similar to fluoxetine.
- **Notes:**
  - Light therapy was shown to be as efficacious as SSRIs in a 2011 Cochrane meta-analysis.

PRACTICE

MDD treatment is gradually escalated when current therapy does not achieve remission.

Evidence

- **Source:** STAR*D Trial. Rush AJ, Trivedi MH, Wisniewski SR, et al. Acute and longer-term outcomes in depressed outpatients requiring one or several treatment steps: a STAR*D report. *Am J Psychiatry.* 2006;163(11):1905–17.
- **Takeaways:**
  - Remission rates of 36.8%, 30.6%, 13.7%, and 13% for the first through fourth treatment steps
  - Requirement for more treatment steps correlated with higher relapse rates
- **Notes:**
  - With bupropion as part of the second-tier strategy, its efficacy was indirectly supported by remission rates.

PRACTICE

In suicidal patients, lithium reduces the risk of suicide.

Evidence

- **Source:** Cipriani A, Hawton K, Stockton S, Geddes JR. Lithium in the prevention of suicide in mood disorders: updated systematic review and meta-analysis. *BMJ.* 2013;346:f3646.
- **Takeaways:**
  - Lithium reduced the rate of suicides (odds ratio [OR] 0.13) and had a mortality benefit (OR 0.38) in patients with mood disorders.
- **Notes:**
  - Acute lithium toxicity may present as cerebellar dysfunction (nystagmus, ataxia) as well as renal toxicity.

PRACTICE

Electroconvulsive therapy (ECT) is a great alternative therapy for MDD particularly in medication-resistant cases.

Evidence

- **Source:** Folkerts HW, Michael N, Tölle R, et al. Electroconvulsive therapy vs. paroxetine in treatment-resistant depression—a randomized study. *Acta Psychiatr Scand.* 1997;96(5):334–42.
- **Takeaways:**
  - ECT was superior to SSRIs in reducing depressive symptoms in medication-refractory patients.
  - The speed of response of ECT was superior.
- **Notes:**
  - Failure to respond to adequate pharmacological treatment for major depression is now the most common indication for the use of ECT.

Bipolar Disorder

PRACTICE

Lithium is a commonly used mood stabilizer in bipolar disorder.

Evidence

- **Source:** Baldessarini RJ, Tondo L. Does lithium treatment still work? Evidence of stable responses over three decades. *Arch Gen Psychiatry.* 2000;57:187–90.
- **Takeaways:**
  - Numerous trials have demonstrated the efficacy of lithium in acute mania though the older trials were less rigorously designed.
  - Newer trials are small but support the findings of earlier trials.
- **Notes:**
  - Lithium was the first medication for bipolar disorder.
  - Lithium takes 4 to 5 days to reach a steady state after starting.
  - Target lithium range is 0.8 to 1.2 mEq/L; levels should be frequently monitored.
  - Once-daily dosing results in higher steady-state levels than BID dosing.
  - Do not take during pregnancy—may cause Ebstein anomaly.

PRACTICE

Valproic acid is a first-line mood stabilizer for bipolar disorder, both as acute and maintenance therapy.

Evidence

- **Source:** Bowden CL, Calabrese JR, McElroy SL, et al. A randomized, placebo-controlled 12-month trial of divalproex and lithium in treatment of outpatients with bipolar I disorder. Divalproex Maintenance Study Group. *Arch Gen Psychiatry.* 2000;57(5):481–9.
- **Takeaways:**
  - Valproate was similar to lithium for time to recurrence of a mood episode.
  - Valproate was superior to lithium for time to a manic or depressive episode and continued treatment duration (198 vs. 152 days).
- **Source:** Bowden CL, Mosolov S, Hranov L, et al. Efficacy of valproate versus lithium in mania or mixed mania: a randomized, open 12-week trial. *Int Clin Psychopharmacol.* 2010;25(2):60–7.
- **Takeaways:**
  - Valproate and lithium had comparable efficacy in treatment of acute mania over 12 weeks.
- **Notes:**
  - Valproate has anti-metabolite properties and should be supplemented with folic acid. High risk for neural tube defects if taken during pregnancy.

PRACTICE

Antidepressants are not recommended as adjunctive therapy in bipolar depression when patients fail mood stabilizer monotherapy.

Evidence

- **Source:** STEP-BD Trial. Sachs GS, Nierenberg AA, Calabrese JR, et al. Effectiveness of adjunctive antidepressant treatment for bipolar depression. *N Engl J Med.* 2007;356(17):1711–22.

- **Takeaways:**
  - Adjunctive antidepressant use was not associated with increased efficacy for bipolar depression.
  - No increase in treatment-emergent affective switch
- **Notes:**
  - Despite the lack of recommendations, it is common for patients to trial antidepressants when mood stabilizer therapy is insufficient.

PRACTICE

Though benzodiazepines are commonly given to bipolar patients, they may impact relapse and should be used judiciously.

Evidence

- **Source:** Perlis RH, Ostacher MJ, Miklowitz DJ, et al. Benzodiazepine use and risk of recurrence in bipolar disorder: a STEP-BD report. *J Clin Psychiatry*, 2010;71(2):194–200.
- **Takeaways:**
  - Benzodiazepine use was associated with higher risk (hazard ratio 1.21) of relapse in bipolar I/II.
- **Notes:**
  - Prospective data was from the STEP-BD study.
  - Benzodiazepine use may be a marker for more severe bipolar disease.

Psychosis

PRACTICE

Second-generation antipsychotics are routinely prescribed for management of psychosis.

Evidence

- **Source:** CATIE Trial. Lieberman JA, Stroup TS, McEvoy JP, et al.; Clinical Antipsychotic Trials of Intervention Effectiveness (CATIE) Investigators. Effectiveness of antipsychotic drugs in patients with chronic schizophrenia. *N Engl J Med.* 2005;353:1209–23.
- **Takeaways:**
  - The time to discontinuation of therapy was significantly longer for olanzapine compared to quetiapine or risperidone.
  - Olanzapine was associated with greater metabolic complications (hyperglycemia, hyperlipidemia, weight gain).
  - No decrease in tardive dyskinesia risk among the second-generation antipsychotics.
- **Notes:**
  - Results are largely consistent with other trials supporting the efficacy of second-generation antipsychotics though not as crystal clear as we would want.
  - A very significant side effect of second-generation antipsychotics are metabolic effects, such as weight gain and increased lipid profiles—regular metabolic monitoring is essential.

PRACTICE

Atypical antipsychotics are not recommended for dementia-associated psychosis, agitation, or aggression, such as in Alzheimer disease.

Evidence

- **Source:** CATIE-AD Trial. Schneider LS, Tariot PN, Dagerman KS, et al. Effectiveness of atypical antipsychotic drugs in patients with Alzheimer's disease. *N Engl J Med.* 2006;355(15):1525–38.
- **Takeaways:**
  - No significant improvement in cognitive ability with atypical antipsychotic therapy
  - Minor trend toward improvement with atypical antipsychotics but outweighed by adverse effects
    - Olanzapine (32%)/quetiapine (26%)/risperidone (29%) versus placebo (21%)
- **Notes:**
  - Key emerging side effects of atypical antipsychotics in dementia include cerebrovascular events and increased mortality.

PRACTICE

Clozapine is a very potent second-generation antipsychotic typically reserved for psychosis refractory to other antipsychotics.

Evidence

- **Source:** Essali A, Al-Haj Haasan N, Li C, Rathbone J. Clozapine versus typical neuroleptic medication for schizophrenia. *Cochrane Database Syst Rev.* 2009;1:CD000059.
- **Takeaways:**
  - Clozapine was associated with more frequent clinical improvement though no difference in mortality.
  - Clozapine led to fewer relapses than typical antipsychotics (RR 0.62).
  - Clozapine demonstrated significantly greater efficacy in patients who had been refractory to other antipsychotics (34% of patients with treatment resistance had clinical improvement).
- **Notes:**
  - Clozapine requires very close monitoring of white blood count for several months after initiation given the risk of agranulocytosis (early symptoms include infectious type such as sore throat).
  - Clozapine is particularly useful for patients with co-occurring suicidal ideation.

Delirium

PRACTICE

The role of antipsychotics in treating delirium in critically ill ICU patients is unclear.

Evidence

- **Source:** MIND-USA Trial. Girard TD, Exline MC, Carson SS, et al. Haloperidol and ziprasidone for treatment of delirium in critical illness. *N Engl J Med.* 2018;379:2506–16.
- **Takeaways:**
  - Haloperidol and ziprasidone did not decrease duration of delirium or coma in critically ill ICU patients.
- **Notes:**
  - Antipsychotics are better at treating hyperactive delirium.
  - This study included largely hypoactive delirium patients.

Alcohol Withdrawal

PRACTICE

The Clinical Institute Withdrawal Assessment (CIWA-Ar) is a commonly used tool to assess symptoms that correlate with alcohol withdrawal.

Evidence

- **Source:** Sullivan JT, Sykora K, Schneiderman J, et al. Assessment of alcohol withdrawal: the revised clinical institute withdrawal assessment for alcohol scale (CIWA-Ar). *Br J Addict.* 1989;84(11):1353–7.
- **Source:** Reoux JP, Miller K. Routine hospital alcohol detoxification practice compared to symptom triggered management with an Objective Withdrawal Scale (CIWA-Ar). *Am J Addict.* 2000;9(2):135–44.
- **Takeaways:**
  - Compared to the full version, the shortened 10-item scale CIWA-Ar had shorter hospitalizations and quantity of benzodiazepine administered.
- **Notes:**
  - CIWA ≤ 8 usually does not require pharmacologic support.

PRACTICE

Benzodiazepine should be used judiciously in alcohol withdrawal with close attention to CIWA. scoring.

Evidence

- **Source:** Daeppen JB, Gache P, Landry U, et al. Symptom-triggered vs. fixed-schedule doses of benzodiazepine for alcohol withdrawal. *Arch Intern Med.* 2003;162(10):1117–21.
- **Takeaways:**
  - Symptom-triggered administration was associated with decreased duration of treatment (20 vs. 62.7 hours for oxazepam treatment duration) and medication quantity (37.5 vs. 231.4 mg).
- **Notes:**
  - Symptoms were quantified by the CIWA scale.
  - It is important to avoid both over-prescribing as well as under-prescribing, therefore highlighting the importance of utilizing as objective a scale as possible (e.g., CIWA).

PRACTICE

Thiamine (Vit B1) is administered prior to glucose when thiamine deficiency is possible (e.g., alcohol abuse) to prevent iatrogenic Wernicke encephalopathy.

Evidence

- **Source:** Schabelman E, Kuo D. Glucose before thiamine for Wernicke encephalopathy: a literature review. *J Emerg Med.* 2012;42(4):488–94.
- **Takeaways:**
  - Glucose administration without thiamine can lead to increased risk for Wernicke encephalopathy though no clear studies are available.
- **Notes:**
  - All evidence based on case reports/series

Vascular Medicine and Surgery

Venous Thromboembolism

PRACTICE

The Wells' Criteria is a commonly used scoring system to determine pulmonary embolism (PE) risk and workup.

Evidence

- **Source:** Wells PS, Anderson DR, Rodger M, et al. Excluding pulmonary embolism at the bedside without diagnostic imaging: management of patients with suspected pulmonary embolism presenting to the emergency department by using a simple clinical model and d-dimer. *Ann Intern Med.* 2001;135(2):98–107.
- **Takeaways:**
  - The Wells' Criteria stratification of PE risk into low, moderate, and high with subsequent management, including D-dimer testing, was safe and decreased need for diagnostic imaging.
- **Notes:**
  - Wells' Criteria Three-Tier Model
    - Low risk (<2 points) = 1.3% PE risk
    - Moderate risk (2 to 6 points) = 16.2% PE risk
    - High risk (>6 points) = 37.5% PE risk

PRACTICE

The pulmonary embolism rule-out criteria (PERC) rule is a scoring system to evaluate the need for D-dimer in low-risk patients stratified by Wells' Criteria.

Evidence

- **Source:** Kline JA, Mitchell AM, Kabrhel C, et al. Clinical criteria to prevent unnecessary diagnostic testing in emergency department patients with suspected pulmonary embolism. *J Thromb Haemost.* 2004;2(8):1247–55.
- **Takeaways:**
  - 96% and 100% sensitive for PE in low-risk and very low-risk populations
- **Source:** Kline JA, Courtney DM, Kabrhel C, et al. Prospective multicenter evaluation of the pulmonary embolism rule-out criteria. *J Thromb Haemost.* 2008;6(5):772–80.

- **Takeaways:**
    - PERC score of 0 with low clinical suspicion had 97.4% sensitivity for PE.
- **Notes:**
    - PERC is only useful in patients low risk for PE.

PRACTICE

In patients greater than 50 years old, D-dimer cutoffs are adjusted for age.

Evidence

- **Source:** ADJUST-PE Trial. Righini M, Van Es J, Exter PLD, et al. Age-adjusted D-dimer cutoff levels to rule out pulmonary embolism: the ADJUST-PE study. *JAMA.* 2014;311(11):1117–24.
- **Takeaways:**
    - 0.1% failure rate of D-dimer in patients with D-dimer greater than 500 µg/L but less than age-adjusted cutoff (age * 10 for patients >50 years)
- **Notes:**
    - Common factors that increase D-dimer levels are renal failure, infection, and obesity.

PRACTICE

CT angiography is the most common diagnostic modality for suspected PE.

Evidence

- **Source:** PIOPED II Trial. Stein PD, Fowler SE, Goodman LR, et al. Multidetector computed tomography for acute pulmonary embolism. *N Engl J Med.* 2006;354:2317–27.
- **Takeaways:**
    - CT angiogram was 96% specific and 83% sensitive for the detection of acute PE.
- **Notes:**
    - Alternative to CTA is V/Q scan (most often used when contraindication to contrast)

PRACTICE

Apixaban is a reasonable first-line choice for anticoagulation in the setting of acute venous thromboembolism (VTE).

Evidence

- **Source:** AMPLIFY Trial. Agnelli G, Buller HR, Cohen A, et al. Oral apixaban for the treatment of acute venous thromboembolism. *N Engl J Med.* 2013;369(9):799–808.
- **Takeaways:**
    - Apixaban was non-inferior to warfarin in treatment of acute VTE.
    - Apixaban was associated with significantly decreased (0.6% vs. 1.8%) major bleeding risk.
- **Notes:**
    - Conventional treatment was either enoxaparin or warfarin.
    - Direct oral anticoagulants offer ease of use (no INR checks) at the expense of reversibility ease.

PRACTICE

Rivaroxaban is a reasonable first-line choice for anticoagulation in the setting of acute VTE.

Evidence

- **Source:** EINSTEIN-DVT Trial. The EINSTEIN Investigators. Oral rivaroxaban for symptomatic venous thromboembolism. *N Engl J Med.* 2010;363:2499–510.
- **Takeaways:**
  - Rivaroxaban was non-inferior to enoxaparin low-molecular-weight heparin (LMWH) in preventing recurrent VTE.
  - No significant difference in bleeding
- **Notes:**
  - No bridging needed
  - Rivaroxaban is convenient to use with once-daily dosing (as opposed to twice daily apixaban).

PRACTICE

Rivaroxaban is a reasonable first-line choice for anticoagulation in the setting of acute PE.

Evidence

- **Source:** EINSTEIN-PE Trial. EINSTEIN-PE Investigators; Büller HR, Prins MH, Lensin AWA, et al. Oral rivaroxaban for the treatment of symptomatic pulmonary embolism. *N Engl J Med.* 2012;366(14):1287–97.
- **Takeaways:**
  - Rivaroxaban was non-inferior to warfarin for initial and long-term treatment of PE.
  - Major bleeding risk tended to favor rivaroxaban (1.1% vs. 2.2%).
- **Notes:**
  - One of the first trials to not utilize an LMWH bridge—Calisto Program (open label pharmacotherapy)

PRACTICE

Dabigatran is a reasonable first-line choice for anticoagulation in the setting of acute VTE.

Evidence

- **Source:** RE-COVER Trial. Schulman S, Kearon C, Kakkar AK, et al.; RE-COVER Study Group. Dabigatran versus warfarin in the treatment of acute venous thromboembolism. *N Engl J Med.* 2009;361(24):2342–52.
- **Takeaways:**
  - Dabigatran 150 mg BID was as effective as warfarin in preventing recurrent VTE and related death.
- **Notes:**
  - Dabigatran does not require routine monitoring.

PRACTICE

Patients who can be treated with anticoagulation for acute proximal deep venous thromboembolism (DVT) do not receive inferior vena cava (IVC) filters for reducing occurrence of PE.

Evidence

- **Source:** PREPIC Trial. Decousus H, Leizorovicz A, Parent F, et al. A clinical trial of vena caval filters in the prevention of pulmonary embolism in patients with proximal deep-vein thrombosis. Prévention du Risque d'Embolie Pulmonaire par Interruption Cave Study Group. *N Engl J Med*. 1998;338:409–16.

- **Takeaways:**
  - No difference in mortality with IVC filter addition
  - Initial benefit (4% absolute reduction) of IVC filters for prevention of pulmonary embolism balanced by excess recurrent DVTs
  - LMWH non-inferior to unfractionated heparin for prevention of pulmonary embolism
- **Notes:**
  - IVC filters are mainly considered for patients with absolute contraindications to anticoagulation or recurrent PE despite anticoagulation.
  - IVC filters may actually increase DVT risk.

PRACTICE

Patients who are treated with anticoagulation for PE do not receive additional IVC filters for reducing occurrence of PE, even if high risk for recurrence.

Evidence

- **Source:** PREPIC2 Trial. Mismetti P, Laporte S, Pellerin O, et al.; PREPIC2 Study Group. Effect of a retrievable inferior vena cava filter plus anticoagulation vs anticoagulation alone on risk of recurrent pulmonary embolism: a randomized clinical trial. *JAMA*. 2015;313(16):1627–35.
- **Takeaways:**
  - No risk reduction (recurrence in three vs. two patients) with IVC addition to anticoagulation
- **Notes:**
  - IVC filters have gradually fallen out of favor except in absolute contraindications to anticoagulation with very high PE risk.
  - IVC filters are difficult to retrieve, particularly if left for a prolonged period.

PRACTICE

LMWH is first-line therapy for DVT/PE in the setting of cancer.

Evidence

- **Source:** CLOT Trial. Lee AY, Levine MN, Baker RI, et al. Low-molecular-weight heparin versus a coumarin for the prevention of recurrent venous thromboembolism in patients with cancer. *N Engl J Med*. 2003;349(2):146–53.
- **Takeaways:**
  - LMWH led to a ~7% absolute reduction in VTE occurrence compared to warfarin in patients with cancer.
  - No difference in bleeding risk between LMWH and warfarin
- **Notes:**
  - Dalteparin was the specific LMWH used.

PRACTICE

Apixaban may be beneficial for reducing VTE in patients with cancer at intermediate-high risk for VTE.

Evidence

- **Source:** AVERT Trial. Carrier M, Abou-Nassar K, Mallick R, et al.; AVERT Investigators. Apixaban to prevent venous thromboembolism in patients with cancer. *N Engl J Med.* 2019;380:711–9.
- **Takeaways:**
  - Compared to placebo, apixaban resulted in significantly less (4.2% vs. 10.2%) VTE.
  - Increased risk of major bleeding with apixaban (3.5% vs. 1.8%)
- **Notes:**
  - Trial focused on patients with cancer due to start chemotherapy, another hit in Virchow triad

PRACTICE

Aspirin may be recommended in patients with unprovoked VTE who have stopped or are to stop anticoagulation.

Evidence

- **Source:** ASPIRE Trial. Brighton TA, Eikelboom JW, Mann K, et al.; ASPIRE Investigators. Low-dose aspirin for preventing recurrent venous thromboembolism. *N Engl J Med.* 2012;367(21):1979–87.
- **Takeaways:**
  - Aspirin 100 mg significantly decreased rate of major vascular events (5.2% vs. 8.0%).
  - Aspirin had a trend toward decreased VTE.
  - No increased bleeding risk with aspirin
- **Source:** WARFASA Trial. Becattini C, Agnelli G, Schenone A, et al.; WARFASA Investigators. Aspirin for preventing the recurrence of venous thromboembolism. *N Engl J Med.* 2012;366(21):1959–67.
- **Takeaways:**
  - Aspirin 100 mg decreased VTE recurrence (6.6% vs. 11.2%) in patients who had discontinued anticoagulation.
  - No significant increase in bleeding with aspirin use
- **Notes:**
  - In the INSPIRE study, results of the ASPIRE and WARFASA trials were combined to show a significant reduction in VTE with aspirin without increasing major bleeding risk.

PRACTICE

Apixaban is reasonable for long-term anticoagulation in patients with VTE.

Evidence

- **Source:** AMPLIFY-EXT Trial. Agnelli G, Buller HR, Cohen A, et al.; AMPLIFY-EXT Investigators. Apixaban for extended treatment of venous thromboembolism. *N Engl J Med.* 2013;368(8):699–708.
- **Takeaways:**
  - Long-term (12 months) apixaban after initial anticoagulation therapy reduced rate of recurrent VTE (1.7% vs. 8.8%).
  - No significant increase in major bleeding events
- **Notes:**
  - Both 2.5 and 5.0 mg doses resulted in the same primary outcome.

PRACTICE

In patients with low to moderate bleeding risk and without reversible risk factors for VTE, rivaroxaban is a reasonable first-line choice for long-term anticoagulation to prevent recurrent VTE after initial anticoagulation for 6 to 12 months.

Evidence

- **Source:** EINSTEIN CHOICE Trial. Weitz JI, Lensing AWA, Prins MH, et al.; EINSTEIN CHOICE Investigators. Rivaroxaban or aspirin for extended treatment of venous thromboembolism. *N Engl J Med.* 2017;376(13):1211–22.
- **Takeaways:**
  - Rivaroxaban 10 mg QD and 20 mg QD both significantly decreased rate of recurrent VTE (1.2% and 1.5% vs. 4.4%, respectively).
  - No significant difference in bleeding compared to aspirin arm
- **Notes:**
  - This study followed patients on average for up to 1 year on rivaroxaban.

PRACTICE

In patients with first time unprovoked VTE, anticoagulation is currently recommended to continue beyond 3 months if the patient is low to moderate bleeding risk while high bleeding risk merits only 3 months. There is some push to investigate ways of risk stratification (such as via D-dimer) to help with determining optimal duration of anticoagulation.

Evidence

- **Source:** DODS Trial. Kearon C, Parpia S, Spencer FA, et al. Long-term risk of recurrence in patients with a first unprovoked venous thromboembolism managed according to D-dimer results; a cohort study. *J Thromb Haemost.* 2019;17(7):1144–52.
- **Takeaways:**
  - VTE recurrence risk was much lower in women than men (17% vs. 29.7%) when anticoagulation was stopped based on a negative D-dimer.
- **Notes:**
  - This study raises the question of incorporating sex into risk stratification methods.

PRACTICE

Continuance of anticoagulation is recommended for patients with recent VTE who have elevated D-dimer levels at the end of their initial anticoagulation course.

Evidence

- **Source:** PROLONG Trial. Palareti G, Cosmi B, Legnani C, et al.; PROLONG Investigators. D-dimer testing to determine the duration of anticoagulation therapy. *N Engl J Med.* 2006;355(17):1780–9.
- **Takeaways:**
  - Elevated D-dimer 1 month after completing initial anticoagulation for VTE was correlated with increased risk (15% vs. 2.9%) for recurrent VTE.
- **Notes:**
  - It is unclear how long patients should remain on anticoagulation for elevated D-dimer levels.

PRACTICE

Thrombolysis in addition to anticoagulation may be carefully considered in select patients with submassive PE.

Evidence

- **Source:** MOPETT Trial. Sharifi M, Bay C, Skrocki L, et al.; "MOPETT" Investigators. Moderate pulmonary embolism treated with thrombolysis. *Am J Cardiol.* 2013;111(2): 273–7.
- **Takeaways:**
  - Low-dose tPA added to anticoagulation markedly decreased pulmonary hypertension or recurrent PE (16% vs. 63%).
  - Open-label single-center
  - Moderate PE definition differed from classic definition for submassive PE.
- **Source:** PEITHO Trial. Meyer G, Vicaut E, Danays T, et al.; PEITHO Investigators. Fibrinolysis for patients with intermediate-risk pulmonary embolism. *N Engl J Med.* 2014;370(15):1402–11.
- **Takeaways:**
  - In submassive PE, fibrinolysis with tenecteplase reduced (1.6% vs. 5.0%) hemodynamic decompensation at 1 week.
  - Increased major bleeding (6.3% vs. 1.2%) and stroke (2.4% vs. 0.2%) risk with fibrinolysis
- **Notes:**
  - No current guidelines recommend routine fibrinolysis for submassive PE.

PRACTICE

Catheter-directed thrombolysis is not recommended to reduce post-thrombotic syndrome rates in patients with acute proximal lower extremity DVT.

Evidence

- **Source:** ATTRACT Trial. Vedantham S, Goldhaber SZ, Julian JA, et al. Pharmacomechanical catheter-directed thrombolysis for deep-vein thrombosis. *N Engl J Med.* 2017;377(23):2240–52.
- **Takeaways:**
  - Compared to anticoagulation alone, pharmacomechanical catheter-directed thrombolysis did not reduce risk of post-thrombotic syndrome.
  - Higher major bleeding risk
- **Notes:**
  - ~50% of DVTs lead to development of post-thrombotic syndrome.

PRACTICE

Patients with a first unprovoked VTE do not merit extensive imaging beyond routine screening recommendations.

Evidence

- **Source:** SOME Trial. Carrier M, Lazo-Langner A, Shivakumar S, et al.; SOME Investigators. Screening for occult cancer in unprovoked venous thromboembolism. *N Engl J Med.* 2015;373(8):697–704.

- **Takeaways:**
  - Low prevalence (3.9%) of occult malignancy in patients with first time unprovoked DVT
  - CT abdomen/pelvis did not increase detection of occult malignancy.
  - No decrease in cancer-related mortality
- **Notes:**
  - The biggest risk factor for VTE is a prior VTE.

Carotid Stenosis

PRACTICE

Aspirin is recommended for all patients undergoing carotid endarterectomy, starting before the surgery and continuing indefinitely.

Evidence

- **Source:** ACE Trial. Taylor DW, Barnett HJ, Haynes RB, et al. Low-dose and high-dose acetylsalicylic acid for patients undergoing carotid endarterectomy: a randomised controlled trial. ASA and Carotid Endarterectomy (ACE) Trial Collaborators. *Lancet.* 1999;353(9171):2179–84.
- **Takeaways:**
  - Low-dose aspirin had a lower risk (5.4% vs. 7.0%) of stroke, MI, or death within 30 days than high-dose aspirin.
- **Notes:**
  - Clopidogrel can be used for aspirin allergies.

PRACTICE

Carotid endarterectomy (CEA) is recommended for symptomatic patients with greater than 70% carotid artery stenosis and asymptomatic patients with greater than 80% carotid artery stenosis.

Evidence

- Symptomatic Patients
  - **Source:** NASCET Trial. Barnett HJ, Taylor DW, Eliasziw M, et al. Benefit of carotid endarterectomy in patients with symptomatic moderate or severe stenosis. North American Symptomatic Carotid Endarterectomy Trial Collaborators. *N Engl J Med.* 1998;339(20):1415–25.
  - **Takeaways:**
    - CEA reduced the 5-year risk of death or stroke by 29% for carotid stenosis greater than 50%.
    - Severe stenosis ≥70% had a significant reduction in stroke at 8 years follow-up.
    - No significant benefit for stenosis less than 50%
  - **Source:** ECST Trial. ECST Group. Randomised trial of endarterectomy for recently symptomatic carotid stenosis: final results of the MRC European Carotid Surgery Trial (ECST). *Lancet.* 1998;351(9113):1379–87.
  - **Takeaways:**
    - CEA significantly reduced mortality and recurrent stroke rates (14.9% vs. 26.5%) in carotid stenosis ≥ 80%.
  - **Source:** North American Symptomatic Carotid Endarterectomy Trial Collaborators. Beneficial effect of carotid endarterectomy in symptomatic patients with high-grade carotid stenosis. *N Engl J Med.* 1991;325:445–53.
  - **Takeaways:**
    - Among severe stenosis (≥70%), 17% absolute risk reduction in ipsilateral stroke

- Asymptomatic Patients
  - **Source:** ACAS Trial. Walker MD, Marler JR, Goldstein M, et al. Endarterectomy for asymptomatic carotid artery stenosis. *JAMA*. 1995;273(18):1421–8.
  - **Takeaways:**
    - Initial study that demonstrated that asymptomatic patients with stenoses greater than 60% had a lower 5-year stroke risk with CEA
  - **Source:** ACST Trial. Halliday A, Harrison M, Hayter E, et al.; Asymptomatic Carotid Surgery Trial (ACST) Collaborative Group. 10-year stroke prevention after successful carotid endarterectomy for asymptomatic stenosis (ACST-1): a multicentre randomised trial. *Lancet*. 2010;376(9746):1074–84.
  - **Takeaways:**
    - In asymptomatic patients less than 75 years old, CEA performed with a cutoff of 60% stenosis significantly reduced 10-year stroke risk.
- **Notes:**
  - Many experts believe that the benefits and risks of CEA highly depend on surgical skill.
  - Difference between stenosis degree required to benefit between trials may be related to different methods of measuring the stenoses. The criteria have evolved often and continue to evolve rapidly.

PRACTICE

Carotid endarterectomy is preferred versus transfemoral carotid artery stenting. Transfemoral carotid artery stenting should largely be performed in patients who are at high anatomic and high medical risk for carotid endarterectomy. It is generally accepted that carotid endarterectomy carries a higher risk of perioperative myocardial infarction, while carotid artery stenting carries a higher risk of perioperative stroke.

Evidence

- **Source:** EVA-3S Trial. Mas JL, Chatellier G, Beyssen B, et al.; EVA-3S Investigators. Endarterectomy versus stenting in patients with symptomatic severe carotid stenosis. *N Engl J Med*. 2006;355:1660–71.
- **Takeaways:**
  - Significantly greater risk of stroke or mortality (relative risk 2.5) with stenting versus endarterectomy for stenosis ≥ 60%
- **Source:** CREST Trial. Brott TG, Hobson RW 2nd, Howard G, et al.; CREST Investigators. Stenting versus endarterectomy for treatment of carotid-artery stenosis. *N Engl J Med*. 2010;363(1):11–23.
- **Takeaways:**
  - No difference between CEA and stenting for stroke, myocardial infarction, or mortality at 4 years
  - Stenting associated with lower periprocedural rates of myocardial infarction
  - CEA associated with lower periprocedural rates of stroke
- **Notes:**
  - CEA carries a higher risk of cranial nerve damage and systemic (pulmonary complications) but differences have not been found to be statistically significant.
  - CEA is associated with greater myocardial infarction while stenting is associated with greater stroke.
  - Future trials include CREST-2, looking at carotid revascularization with carotid artery stenting vs. CEA vs. medical management only (currently suspended due to COVID-19).

PRACTICE

Eversion carotid endarterectomy is a reasonable method of performing CEA for carotid stenosis, largely for patients with redundant ICAs to prevent further tortuosity and/or kinking.

Evidence

- **Source:** EVEREST Trial. Cao P, Giordano G, De Rango P, et al. A randomized study on eversion versus standard carotid endarterectomy: study design and preliminary results: the Everest Trial. *J Vasc Surg.* 1998;27(4):595–605.
- **Takeaways:**
  - No difference in restenosis rates between eversion and standard CEA
  - Eversion CEA is safe and has low complication rates.

PRACTICE

The ENROUTE Transcarotid Neuroprotection System is used by many vascular surgeons as a way to reduce the risk of stroke during carotid artery stenting.

Evidence

- **Source:** ROADSTER Trial. Kwolek CJ, Jaff MR, Leal JI, et al. Results of the ROADSTER multicenter trial of transcarotid stenting with dynamic flow reversal. *J Vasc Surg.* 2015;62(5):1227–34.
- **Takeaways:**
  - Stroke rate of 1.4% (lowest in any study) for carotid stenting performed on a mixture of symptomatic and asymptomatic patients

Peripheral Arterial Disease

PRACTICE

A supervised exercise regimen is first-line therapy for peripheral arterial disease (PAD).

Evidence

- **Source:** CLEVER Trial. Murphy TP, Cutlip DE, Regensteiner JG, et al.; CLEVER Study Investigators. Supervised exercise versus primary stenting for claudication resulting from aortoiliac peripheral artery disease. *Circulation.* 2012;125:130–9.
- **Takeaways:**
  - Supervised exercise was superior to stenting for improving walking performance.
- **Notes:**
  - 6-minute walking outcomes not tracked in this study

PRACTICE

For maximal symptomatic and functional relief, patients with peripheral artery disease (PAD) may be considered for endovascular revascularization on top of a supervised exercise regimen.

Evidence

- **Source:** ERASE Trial. Fakhry F, Spronk S, van der Laan L, et al. Endovascular revascularization and supervised exercise for peripheral artery disease and intermittent claudication: a randomized clinical trial. *JAMA.* 2015;314(18):1936–44.

- **Takeaways:**
  - Combination of endovascular revascularization with supervised exercise resulted in better walking distance and quality of life measures
- **Notes:**
  - Walking was measured with treadmill walking distance (not 6-minute walk test).

PRACTICE

Cilostazol is recommended for symptomatic management of intermittent claudication in peripheral arterial disease.

Evidence

- **Source:** Dawson DL, Cutler BS, Meissner MH, Strandness DE Jr. Cilostazol has beneficial effects in treatment of intermittent claudication: results from a multicenter, randomized, prospective, double blind trial. *Circulation.* 1998;98(7).678–86.
- **Takeaways:**
  - Cilostazol significantly improved (35% increase in initial claudication distance, 41% increase in absolute claudication distance) walking distance compared to placebo.
- **Notes:**
  - Cilostazol acts as a phosphodiesterase inhibitor, dilating arteries and suppressing platelet aggregation.
  - BASIL-2 and BEST-CLI are ongoing trials to further investigate the best management for PAD, which still remains controversial.

PRACTICE

Patients with severe PAD resulting in leg ischemia are favored to undergo open bypass revascularization.

Evidence

- **Source:** BASIL Trial. Bradbury AW, Adam DJ, Bell J, et al.; BASIL Trial Participants. Bypass versus angioplasty in severe ischaemia of the leg (BASIL) trial: analysis of amputation free and overall survival by treatment received. *J Vasc Surg.* 2010;51(5):A1–12.
- **Takeaways:**
  - Angioplasty was associated with a significantly higher early failure rate than open bypass surgery.
  - Most angioplasty patients ultimately required open surgery.
- **Notes:**
  - BASIL-2 and BEST-CLI are ongoing trials to further investigate the best management for PAD, which remains controversial.

Rheumatology

Rheumatology is another specialty that draws its experience from expert opinion given the dearth of large randomized controlled trials. These studies reflect the more common clinical scenarios clinicians will see.

Ankylosing Spondylitis

PRACTICE

In patients with active ankylosing spondylitis who have an inadequate response to NSAIDs, tumor necrosis factor (TNF) inhibitors are used as a first-choice biologic agent.

Evidence

- **Source:** Brandt J, Khariouzov A, Listing J, et al. Six-month results of a double-blind, placebo-controlled trial of etanercept treatment in patients with active ankylosing spondylitis. *Arthritis Rheum.* 2003 Jun;48(6):1667–75.
- **Takeaways:**
  - In this multi-center, double-blind placebo-controlled trial, patients with active ankylosing spondylitis were either given etanercept or placebo for 6 weeks and were followed up for 24 weeks. Patients in the treatment arm resulted in 50% regression of disease activity in 57% of patients versus 6% in the placebo-treated patients. After the placebo-treated patients switched to etanercept, 56% of them improved. Disease relapses occurred around 6 weeks after cessation of etanercept.
- **Notes:**
  - Contraindications to tumor necrosis factor (TNF) inhibitors include active infection, latent untreated tuberculosis, demyelinating diseases, heart failure, and malignancy.

Dermatomyositis and Polymyositis

PRACTICE

Several categories of autoantibodies can be used to diagnose particular clinical syndromes within the myositis spectrum.

Evidence

- **Source:** Love LA, Leff RL, Fraser DD, et al. A new approach to the classification of idiopathic inflammatory myopathy: myositis-specific autoantibodies define useful homogeneous patient groups. *Medicine (Baltimore)*. 1991;70(6):360–74.
- **Takeaways:**
  - In this study, the group compared the usefulness of myositis-specific autoantibodies (anti-aminoacyl-tRNA synthetases, anti-SRP, anti-Mi-2, and anti-MAS) to the standard clinical categories (polymyositis, dermatomyositis, overlap myositis, cancer-associated myositis, and inclusion body myositis) in predicting clinical signs and symptoms, human leukocyte antigen types, and prognosis in 212 adult patients. They showed that the myositis-specific autoantibodies aid in interpreting the diverse symptoms and signs of myositis patients and in predicting their clinical course and prognosis.
- **Notes:**
  - For example, patients with anti-amino-acyl-tRNA synthetase autoantibodies, when compared to those without these antibodies, had significantly more frequent arthritis, fever, interstitial lung disease, and "mechanic's hands."

Gout

PRACTICE

Patients with gout are advised against eating higher levels of meat and seafood.

Evidence

- **Source:** Choi HK, Atkinson K, Karlson EW, et al. Purine-rich foods, dairy and protein intake, and the risk of gout in men. *N Engl J Med*. 2004;350(11):1093–103.
- **Takeaways:**
  - Over a 12-year period, this study prospectively examined the relationship between dietary risk factors and new cases of gout among 47,150 men who had no history of gout at baseline. 730 new cases of gout were confirmed, and in that population, the multivariate relative risk of gout among men in the highest quintile of meat intake, compared to the lowest quintile, was 1.41. The relative risk associated with seafood intake was 1.51.
- **Notes:**
  - Interestingly, this study also showed that the relative risk associated with dairy between the highest and lowest quintile was 0.56. Thus, increased low-fat dairy consumption is recommended for these patients.

PRACTICE

Patients with gout are advised against drinking excessive alcohol.

Evidence

- **Source:** Choi HK, Atkinson K, Karlson EW, et al. Alcohol intake and risk of incident gout in men: a prospective study. *Lancet*. 2004 Apr 17;363(9417):1277–81.
- **Takeaways:**
  - In this prospective study, they had 730 confirmed new incident cases of gout. Compared with men who did not drink alcohol, the multivariate relative risk (RR) of gout was 1.32 for alcohol consumption 10.0 to 14.9 g/day, 1.49 for 15.0 to 29.9 g/day, 1.96 30.0 to 49.9 g/day, and 2.53 ≥ 50 g/day.

- **Notes:**
  - Additionally, beer consumption showed the strongest independent association with the risk of gout.

PRACTICE

A short-term course of glucocorticoids is used during an acute gout flare.

Evidence

- **Source:** Janssens HJ, Janssen M, van de Lisdonk EH, et al. Use of oral prednisolone or naproxen for the treatment of gout arthritis: a double-blind, randomised equivalence trial. *Lancet.* 2008 May 31;371(9627):1854–60.
- **Takeaways:**
  - In this randomized placebo-controlled trial, 120 patients were assigned to receive either prednisolone or naproxen. The primary outcome was pain measured on a 100 mm visual analogue scale. After 90 hours, reduction in pain score was 44.7 and 46.0 mm for prednisolone and naproxen, respectively.
- **Notes:**
  - In patients where only one or two joints are involved, joint aspiration and injection with a glucocorticoid provide another option.

PRACTICE

Colchicine prophylaxis can be used during initiation of allopurinol for chronic gouty arthritis.

Evidence

- **Source:** Borstad GC, Bryant LR, Abel MP, et al. Colchicine for prophylaxis of acute flares when initiating allopurinol for chronic gouty arthritis. *J Rheumatol.* 2004 Dec;31(12):2429–32.
- **Takeaways:**
  - In this randomized, prospective, double-blind, placebo-controlled trial, patients were assigned to receive colchicine or placebo while they were initiated on allopurinol. The patients in the colchicine arm experienced fewer total flares (0.52 vs. 2.91). Additionally, gout flares were reported to be less severe (based on visual analog scale).
- **Notes:**
  - Colchicine is generally continued for 3 to 6 months after achievement of the goal urate level to prevent gout flares.

PRACTICE

Febuxostat should be reserved for patients who have failed or do not tolerate allopurinol.

Evidence

- **Source:** Schumacher HR Jr, Becker MA, Wortmann RL, et al. Effects of febuxostat versus allopurinol and placebo in reducing serum urate in subjects with hyperuricemia and gout: a 28-week, phase III, randomized, double-blind, parallel-group trial. *Arthritis Rheum.* 2008 Nov 15;59(11):1540–8.
- **Source:** White WB, Saag KG, Becker MA, et al. Cardiovascular safety of febuxostat or allopurinol in patients with gout. *N Engl J Med.* 2018 Mar 29;378(13):1200–10.

- **Takeaways:**
  - In the original randomized, double-blind trial in 2008, patients with hyperuricemia gout with normal or impaired renal function were randomized to receive once-daily febuxostat, allopurinol (300 or 100 mg, based on renal function), or placebo for 28 weeks. Significantly ($P \leq .05$) higher percentages of subjects treated with febuxostat attained the primary end point of last 3 monthly serum urate levels <6.0 mg/dL compared with allopurinol (22%) and placebo (0%).
  - However, this trial did not account for any cardiac complications from this drug. In the 2018 trial, 6190 patients underwent randomization, received febuxostat or allopurinol, and were followed for a median of 32 months. The primary end-point event (cardiovascular death, nonfatal myocardial infarction, nonfatal stroke, or unstable angina) occurred in 335 patients (10.8%) in the febuxostat group and in 321 patients (10.4%) in the allopurinol group. All-cause and cardiovascular mortality were higher in the febuxostat group than in the allopurinol group.
- **Notes:**
  - Febuxostat should be started at 40 mg once daily and titrated to 80 mg daily.

Osteoarthritis

PRACTICE

In patients with osteoarthritis of the knee and obesity, a weight loss regimen through exercise and dieting should be the first step in management.

Evidence

- **Source:** Messier SP, Mihalko SL, Legault C, et al. Effects of intensive diet and exercise on knee joint loads, inflammation, and clinical outcomes among overweight and obese adults with knee osteoarthritis: the IDEA randomized clinical trial. *JAMA.* 2013 Sep 25;310(12):1263–73.
- **Takeaways:**
  - In this single-blind, randomized clinical trial, patients were assigned to either a diet + exercise regimen, diet-only regimen, or exercise-only regimen. Mean weight loss for diet + exercise participants was 10.6 kg (11.4%); for the diet group, 8.9 kg (9.5%); and for the exercise group, 1.8 kg (2.0%). After 18 months, knee compressive forces were lower in diet participants (2487 Newtons) compared with exercise participants (2687 Newtons). Concentrations of interleukin-6 were lower in diet + exercise (2.7 pg/mL) and diet participants (2.7 pg/mL) compared with exercise participants (3.1 pg/mL).
- **Notes:**
  - Pharmacologic agents should be reserved for patients with osteoarthritis who have not responded adequately to initial nonpharmacologic measures.

PRACTICE

In patients with osteoarthritis of the knee and obesity, hyaluronic acid should not be routinely used in the treatment of knee osteoarthritis.

Evidence

- **Source:** Jevsevar D, Donnelly P, Brown GA, Cummins DS. Viscosupplementation for osteoarthritis of the knee: a systematic review of the evidence. *J Bone Joint Surg Am.* 2015;97(24):2047–60.

- **Takeaways:**
  - In this systematic review, this group showed that the most consistent finding was that double-blinded, sham-controlled trials had much smaller treatment effects than trials that were not sufficiently blinded ($P < .05$). For double-blinded trials, the overall treatment effect was less than half of the minimal important difference for pain, function, and stiffness. Overall, the meta-analysis of only the double-blinded, sham-controlled trials with at least 60 patients did not show clinically important differences of hyaluronic acid treatment over placebo.
- **Notes:**
  - It was originally thought that hyaluronic acid may aid in stimulating an increase in the growth of cartilage-producing cells.

PRACTICE

In patients with osteoarthritis of the knee and obesity, platelet-rich plasma (PRP) should not be used as standard of treatment in knee osteoarthritis as it is still currently under investigation.

Evidence

- **Source:** Laudy AB, Bakker EW, Rekers M, Moen MH. Efficacy of platelet-rich plasma injections in osteoarthritis of the knee: a systematic review and meta-analysis. *Br J Sports Med.* 2015;49(10):657–72.
- **Takeaways:**
  - In this systematic review, 10 trials looking at PRP were included. The analysis did show that intra-articular PRP injections were more effective for pain reduction compared with placebo at 6 months postinjection. Intra-articular PRP injections were compared with hyaluronic acid and showed a statistically significant difference in favor of PRP on pain reduction based on the visual analogue scale and numeric rating scale at 6 months postinjection. However, almost all trials revealed a high risk of bias. Thus, more large, randomized studies of good quality and low risk of bias are needed to test whether PRP injections should be a routine part of management of patients with OA of the knee.
- **Notes:**
  - The mechanism of action is not well-understood, but it is thought to provide high concentrations of growth factors including tissue growth factor and platelet-derived growth factors, which can mediate the proliferation of mesenchymal stem cells and increase matrix synthesis and collagen formation.

Rheumatoid Arthritis

PRACTICE

- Methotrexate (MTX) is used as the most common first line agent in the treatment of rheumatoid arthritis (RA).

Evidence

- **Source:** Choi HK, Hernán MA, Seeger JD, et al. Methotrexate and mortality in patients with rheumatoid arthritis: a prospective study. *Lancet.* 2002 Apr 6;359(9313): 1173–7.

- **Takeaways:**
  - In this single-site prospective study, 1240 patients with rheumatoid arthritis compared patients who were prescribed MTX versus those who were not. The mortality hazard ratio for MTX use compared with no MTX use was 0.4. Other conventional disease-modifying antirheumatic drugs did not have a significant effect on mortality. The hazard ratio of MTX use for cardiovascular death was 0.3 whereas that for non-cardiovascular deaths was 0.6.
- **Notes:**
  - MTX is contraindicated in patients who are contemplating becoming pregnant/are pregnant, patients with liver disease, and patients with severe renal impairment.

PRACTICE

- Rituximab is another effective therapy that is used with MTX in patients who have had an inadequate response to anti-TNF therapies.

Evidence

- **Source:** Cohen SB, Emery P, Greenwald MW, et al. Rituximab for rheumatoid arthritis refractory to anti-tumor necrosis factor therapy: results of a multicenter, randomized, double-blind, placebo-controlled, phase III trial evaluating primary efficacy and safety at twenty-four weeks. *Arthritis Rheum.* 2006;54(9):2793–806.
- **Takeaways:**
  - In this clinical trial, patients were assigned to either placebo (*n* = 209) or rituximab (*n* = 311). At week 24, significantly more rituximab-treated patients than placebo-treated patients demonstrated American College of Rheumatology Score (ACR) 20 (51% vs. 18%), ACR 50 (27% vs. 5%), and ACR 70 (12% vs. 1%) responses. All ACR response parameters were significantly improved in rituximab-treated patients, who also had clinically meaningful improvements in fatigue, disability, and health-related quality of living.
  - The rate of serious infections was 5.2 per 100 patient-years in the rituximab group and 3.7 per 100 patient-years in the placebo group.
- **Notes:**
  - Rituximab is a monoclonal anti-CD20 antibody that depletes B cells. It is available for use in Rheumatoid Arthritis (RA), systemic vasculitis, and other rheumatic diseases. It is an important therapeutic agent for the treatment of B-cell malignancies and is used in a number of other disorders.

PRACTICE

- Etanercept can alternatively be used as a first-line agent in early rheumatoid arthritis.

Evidence

- **Source:** Bathon JM, Martin RW, Fleischmann RM, et al. A comparison of etanercept and MTX in patients with early rheumatoid arthritis. *N Engl J Med.* 2000 Nov 30;343(22):1586–93.
- **Takeaways:**
  - In this trial, 632 patients with early rheumatoid arthritis were given either twice-weekly subcutaneous etanercept or weekly oral MTX. As compared with patients who received MTX, patients who received the etanercept had a more rapid rate of improvement, with significantly more patients having improvement in disease activity during

the first 6 months. The mean increase in the erosion score during the first 6 months was 0.30 in the group assigned to receive etanercept and 0.68 in the MTX group, and the respective increases during the first 12 months were 0.47 and 1.03. Among patients who received etanercept, 72% had no increase in the erosion score, as compared with 60% of patients in the MTX group.

- Notes:
  - Etanercept mimics the inhibitory effects of naturally occurring soluble TNF, though has a greatly extended half-life compared to a naturally occurring soluble TNF receptor.

PRACTICE

- Use of abatacept

Evidence

- **Source:** Emery P, Burmester GR, Bykerk VP, et al. Evaluating drug-free remission with abatacept in early rheumatoid arthritis: results from the phase 3b, multicentre, randomised, active-controlled AVERT study of 24 months, with a 12-month, double-blind treatment period. *Ann Rheum Dis.* 2015 Jan;74(1):19–26.
- **Source:** Westhovens R, Robles M, Ximenes AC, et al. Clinical efficacy and safety of abatacept in MTX-naive patients with early rheumatoid arthritis and poor prognostic factors. *Ann Rheum Dis.* 2009 Dec;68(12):1870–7.
- **Takeaways:**
  - In the 2009 trial, patients with early RA and erosive joint changes the combination of abatacept with MTX was superior to MTX alone, but without added safety concerns. In this trial of RA patients with less than 2 years disease duration, a similar proportion of patients receiving abatacept monotherapy and MTX monotherapy achieved clinical remission (Disease Activity Score in 28 joints and the C-reactive protein [DAS28-CRP] <2.6 in 43% and 45%, respectively). The treatments demonstrated similar safety profiles.
- Notes:
  - Abatacept works by preventing antigen-presenting cells from delivering their co-stimulatory signal, thus preventing T cells from being fully activated.

PRACTICE

- Use of tocilizumab

Evidence

- **Source:** Smolen JS, Beaulieu A, Rubbert-Roth A, et al. Effect of interleukin-6 receptor inhibition with tocilizumab in patients with rheumatoid arthritis (OPTION study): a double-blind, placebo-controlled, randomised trial. *Lancet.* 2008 Mar 22;371(9617):987–97.
- **Takeaways:**
  - In this double-blind, randomized, placebo-controlled trial patients were assigned to receive tocilizumab at 8 mg/kg, at 4 mg/kg, or placebo. The primary endpoint was the proportion of patients with 20% improvement in signs and symptoms (ACR20 response) at week 24. ACR20 response was seen in more patients receiving tocilizumab (59% of patients in the 8mg/kg group and 48% in the 4 mg/kg group) compared to just 26% in the placebo group.
- Notes:
  - Tocilizumab works by inhibition of the interleukin-6 receptor to decrease the inflammatory response.

PRACTICE

- In patients with early rheumatoid arthritis, the use of low-dose steroids can be utilized to rapidly minimize disease activity while awaiting a clinical response to a slower-acting disease-modifying antirheumatic drug.

Evidence

- **Source:** Svensson B, Boonen A, Albertsson K, et al. Low-dose prednisolone in addition to the initial disease-modifying antirheumatic drug in patients with early active rheumatoid arthritis reduces joint destruction and increases the remission rate: a two-year randomized trial. *Arthritis Rheum.* 2005 Nov;52(11):3360–70.
- **Takeaways**:
  - In this 2-year randomized trial, patients were started on a disease-modifying antirheumatic drug and were randomly assigned to receive either prednisolone or no prednisolone for 2 years. Radiographs of the hands and feet were obtained at baseline and after 1 and 2 years and scored according to the Sharp score as modified by van der Heijde. At 2 years, the median and interquartile range (IQR) change in total Sharp score was lower in the prednisolone group than in the no prednisolone group (1.8 vs. 3.6). In the prednisolone group, there were fewer newly eroded joints per patient after 2 years. In the prednisolone group, 25.9% of patients had radiographic progression compared with 39.3% of patients in the no prednisolone group. At 2 years, 55.5% of patients in the prednisolone group had achieved disease remission, compared with 32.8% of patients in the no prednisolone group.
- **Notes:**
  - Typically, glucocorticoids are added on for only a short period (1 month or less).

PRACTICE

- In patients with early, severe, rheumatoid arthritis, a combination of MTX + etanercept is effective for disease remission and radiographic non-progression.

Evidence

- **Source:** Emery P, Breedveld FC, Hall S, et al. Comparison of MTX monotherapy with a combination of MTX and etanercept in active, early, moderate to severe rheumatoid arthritis (COMET): a randomised, double-blind, parallel treatment trial. *Lancet.* 2008 Aug 2;372(9636):375–82.
- **Takeaways:**
  - Participants were randomly assigned to either receive combined etanercept + MTX treatment or MTX alone.
  - 132 of 265 (50%) patients who took combined treatment achieved clinical remission compared with 73 of 263 (28%) taking MTX alone.
  - 196 of 246 (80%) in the combined treatment group and 135 of 230 (59%) of the MTX-only group achieved radiographic non-progression.

Scleroderma

PRACTICE

- Cyclophosphamide is used in patients with symptomatic scleroderma-related interstitial lung disease.

Evidence

- **Source:** Tashkin DP, Elashoff R, Clements PJ, et al. Cyclophosphamide versus placebo in scleroderma lung disease. *N Engl J Med.* 2006 Jun 22;354(25):2655–66.
- **Takeaways:**
  - In this multicenter study, scleroderma patients with evidence of interstitial lung disease were randomly assigned to receive either oral cyclophosphamide or matching placebo for 1 year and were followed for an additional year. The adjusted 12-month forced vital capacity (FVC) percent predicted between the cyclophosphamide and placebo groups was 2.53% favoring cyclophosphamide. There were also treatment-related differences in physiological and symptom outcomes, and the difference in FVC was maintained at 24 months.
- **Notes:**
  - Cyclophosphamide is dosed intermittently as compared to daily in order to prevent drug-induced cystitis. Aggressive hydration is advised.

PRACTICE

- Long-acting dihydropyridine calcium channel blockers (CCBs) are used in Raynaud phenomenon when conventional therapies fail.

Evidence

- **Source:** Rodeheffer RJ, Rommer JA, Wigley F, Smith CR. Controlled double-blind trial of nifedipine in the treatment of Raynaud's phenomenon. *N Engl J Med.* 1983 Apr 14;308(15):880–3.
- **Takeaways:**
  - In this prospective study, 15 patients were observed over a 7-week period. During the first 2-week period, each patient received placebo and then were randomly assigned to receive either nifedipine or placebo in a double-blind crossover trial. Moderate to marked improvement was reported by 60% of the patients when they were taking nifedipine and by 13% of the patients when they were taking placebo. The mean attack rate of Raynaud's fell from 14.7 attacks per 2 weeks with placebo to 10.8 attacks per 2 weeks with nifedipine.
- **Notes:**
  - There is no clear data to support the use of one long-acting dihydropyridine CCB over another.

PRACTICE

- Epoprostenol can be used to reduce the number of frequency and duration of attacks of Raynaud crisis. It can also reduce the chance of digital ulcerations in patients with systemic sclerosis.

Evidence

- **Source:** Belch JJ, Newman P, Drury JK, et al. Intermittent epoprostenol (prostacyclin) infusion in patients with Raynaud's syndrome. A double-blind controlled trial. *Lancet.* 1983;1(8320):313–15.
- **Source:** Badesch DB, Tapson VF, McGoon MD, et al. Continuous intravenous epoprostenol for pulmonary hypertension due to the scleroderma spectrum of disease. A randomized, controlled trial. *Ann Intern Med.* 2000;132(6):425–34.

- **Takeaways:**
  - In this study, two groups of patients were randomly allocated to receive at weekly intervals for 3 weeks either a 5-hour intravenous infusion of buffer or epoprostenol (prostacyclin, PGI2) in buffer (7.5 ng/kg/min after the first hour). The patients who received the infusions reduced the frequency and duration of ischemic attacks. In this second study, trends toward greater improvement in severity of the Raynaud phenomenon and fewer new digital ulcers were seen in the epoprostenol group.
- **Notes:**
  - Epoprostenol is currently approved for the treatment of pulmonary arterial hypertension and works as a vasodilator of the pulmonary and systemic vascular beds.

Evidence

- **Source:** Rodeheffer RJ, Rommer JA, Wigley F, Smith CR. Controlled double-blind trial of nifedipine in the treatment of Raynaud's phenomenon. *N Engl J Med.* 1983 Apr 14;308(15):880–3.
- **Takeaways:**
  - In this prospective study, 15 patients were observed over a 7-week period. During the first 2-week period, each patient received placebo and then were randomly assigned to receive either nifedipine or placebo in a double-blind crossover trial. Moderate to marked improvement was reported by 60% of the patients when they were taking nifedipine and by 13% of the patients when they were taking placebo. The mean attack rate of Raynaud's fell from 14.7 attacks per 2 weeks with placebo to 10.8 attacks per 2 weeks with nifedipine.
- **Notes:**
  - There is no clear data to support the use of one long-acting dihydropyridine CCB over another.

Systemic Lupus Erythematosus

PRACTICE

- The 2019 European League Against Rheumatism/American College of Rheumatology classification criteria should be used for the classification for systemic lupus erythematosus (SLE).

Evidence

- **Source:** Aringer M, Costenbader K, Daikh D, et al. 2019 European League Against Rheumatism/American College of Rheumatology classification criteria for systemic lupus erythematosus. *Arthritis Rheumatol.* 2019 Sep;71(9):1400–12.
- **Takeaways:**
  - The 2019 EULAR/ACR classification criteria for SLE include positive antinuclear antibody at least once as obligatory entry criterion, followed by additive weighted criteria grouped in seven clinical (constitutional, hematological, neuropsychiatric, mucocutaneous, serosal, musculoskeletal, renal) and three immunological (antiphospholipid antibodies, complement proteins, SLE-specific antibodies) domains, and weighted from 2 to 10. Patients accumulating ≥10 points are classified. In the validation cohort, the new criteria had a sensitivity of 96.1% and specificity of 93.4%, compared with 82.8% sensitivity and 93.4% specificity of the ACR 1997 and 96.7% sensitivity and 83.7% specificity of the Systemic Lupus International Collaborating Clinics 2012 criteria.

- **Notes:**
  - This criteria provides an improved foundation for SLE research.

PRACTICE

- Hydroxychloroquine is a standard of care SLE therapy.

Evidence

- **Source:** Ruiz-Irastorza G, Ramos-Casals M, Brito-Zeron P, Khamashta MA. Clinical efficacy and side effects of antimalarials in systemic lupus erythematosus: a systematic review. *Ann Rheum Dis.* 2010 Jan;69(1):20–8.
- **Takeaways:** A systematic review of the English literature between 1982 and 2007 was conducted using the MEDLINE and EMBASE databases. Randomized controlled trials (RCTs) and observational studies were selected with a total of 95 articles included in the systematic review. High levels of evidence were found that antimalarials prevent lupus flares and increase long-term survival of patients with SLE and that there was moderate evidence of protection against irreversible organ damage, thrombosis, and bone mass loss.
- **Notes:**
  - The risk of retinal toxicity is less than 1% in patients who have taken hydroxychloroquine for less than 5 years but increases the longer they have been on the medication.

PRACTICE

- Mycophenolate mofetil is noninferior to intravenous cyclophosphamide as induction therapy in lupus nephritis.

Evidence

- **Source:** Ginzler EM, Dooley MA, Aranow C, et al. Mycophenolate mofetil or intravenous cyclophosphamide for lupus nephritis. *N Engl J Med.* 2005 Nov 24;353(21):2219–28.
- **Takeaways:**
  - In this trial, patients were randomly selected to receive mycophenolate mofetil or cyclophosphamide. At 12 weeks, 56 patients receiving mycophenolate mofetil and 42 receiving cyclophosphamide had satisfactory early responses. 22.5% receiving mycophenolate mofetil and 5.8% receiving cyclophosphamide had complete remission.
- **Notes:**
  - A complete blood count (CBC) should be performed 1 to 2 weeks after the start of therapy. If there is no evidence of bone marrow suppression at that time, CBCs can then be checked every 6 to 8 weeks.

PRACTICE

- Mycophenolate mofetil is used for maintaining a renal response to treatment and in preventing relapse in lupus nephritis.

Evidence

- **Source:** Dooley MA, Jayne D, Ginzler EM, et al. Mycophenolate versus azathioprine as maintenance therapy for lupus nephritis. *N Engl J Med.* 2011;365(20):1886–95.

■ **Takeaways**:
  ■ A total of 227 patients were randomly assigned to maintenance treatment to either mycophenolate mofetil or azathioprine. Mycophenolate mofetil was superior to azathioprine with respect to the primary end point, time to treatment failure (hazard ratio 0.4), and with respect to time to renal flare and time to rescue therapy (hazard ratio <1.00). Observed rates of treatment failure were 16.4% in the mycophenolate mofetil group and 32.4% in the azathioprine group.
■ **Notes:**
  ■ Mycophenolate inhibits inosine monophosphate dehydrogenase, leading to decreased B- and T-cell proliferation.

PRACTICE

■ Belimumab is used as a targeted biological treatment that is specifically approved for SLE.

Evidence

■ **Source:** Navarra SV, Guzmán RM, Gallacher AE, et al. Efficacy and safety of belimumab in patients with active systemic lupus erythematosus: a randomised, placebo-controlled, phase 3 trial. *Lancet.* 2011;377(9767):721–31.
■ **Takeaways**:
  ■ In this study, 867 patients were randomly assigned to belimumab 1 mg/kg (n = 289) or 10 mg/kg (n = 290), or placebo (n = 288). Significantly higher Systemic Lupus Erythematosus Responder Index rates were noted with belimumab 1 mg/kg (148 [51%], odds ratio 1.55 [95% CI 1.10 to 2.19]; P = .0129) and 10 mg/kg (167 [58%], 1·83 [1.30 to 2.59]; P = .0006) than with placebo (125 [44%]) at week 52. Rates of adverse events were similar in the groups given belimumab 1 mg/kg and 10 mg/kg, and placebo: serious infection was reported in 22 (8%), 13 (4%), and 17 (6%) patients, respectively.
■ **Notes:**
  ■ *Belimumab* is a fully humanized IgG1γ monoclonal antibody directed against soluble B lymphocyte stimulator, and it was the first biological agent specifically approved for SLE.

Congratulations on finishing your introduction to evidence-based medicine! The following are a few resources you may be interested in to continue developing your skills and stay abreast of the latest developments in medical research.

If you are interested in staying up to date with the latest clinical studies, consider subscribing to the weekly New England Journal of Medicine email newsletters.

Ongoing clinical trials can be searched on clinicaltrials.gov. Here you may search by various parameters such as disease, institution, investigators, funding source, and eligibility criteria. It is a great place to keep abreast of the latest developments in a particular field of medicine.

Lastly, here are a list of resources to further your learning of clinical statistics:
- Medical Statistics: For Beginners by Ramakrishna HK
- Statistics in Medicine by Robert Riffenburgh and Daniel Gillen

Note: Page numbers followed by "f" indicate figures, "b" indicate boxes, and "t" indicate tables.